THREE WOMEN, DIFFERENT LIVES... ONE PROBLEM

Susan. At thirty-seven, married, and with a three-year-old son, she was about twenty pounds overweight, most of it in her stomach and hips. She complained of fatigue, heavy periods, and an inability to get pregnant again. An exam discovered a fibroid tumor on her uterus. Her doctor said she needed surgery...

Anne. A forty-four-year-old schoolteacher, she went to her doctor complaining of weight gain, depression, and headaches. The prescription hormones she was given made her depression worse and her headaches intolerable. When her pap smear revealed cervical dysplasia, her doctor recommended a hysterectom...

Marie. Thin, attractive, and always in motion, the thirty-nine-year-old attorney had night sweats, severe cramps in the middle of her menstrual cycle, and spotty bleeding throughout the month. A minor exploratory surgery uncovered cysts on her ovaries. Her doctor removed one ovary, and yet her symptoms are back...

THESE WOMEN WERE SUFFERING FROM PRE-MENOPAUSE SYNDROME. TODAY THEY ARE SYMPTOM-FREE AND HEALTHY—WITHOUT SURGERY OR PRESCRIPTION HORMONES.

FIND OUT HOW IN...

WHAT YOUR DOCTOR MAY NOT TELL YOU ABOUT™ PREMENOPAUSE

WHAT YOUR DOCTOR MAY NOT TELL YOU ABOUT™

PREMENOPAUSE

Balance Your Hormones and Your Life from Thirty to Fifty

JOHN R. LEE, M.D.,
JESSE HANLEY, M.D., and VIRGINIA HOPKINS
Bestselling authors of *What Your Doctor May Not Tell You About Menopause*

GRAND CENTRAL
PUBLISHING

NEW YORK   BOSTON

Some of the material in this book originally appeared in the *John R. Lee, M.D., Medical Letter.*

Author's note: Unless it is explicitly otherwise stated, the personal details of the experiences shared by women in this book have all been changed so as to protect their identities, but the essential experiences remain the same.

Cover design by Diane Luger

Grand Central Publishing
Hachette Book Group
237 Park Avenue, New York, NY 10017
Visit our Web site at www.HachetteBookGroup.com

Grand Central Publishing is a division of Hachette Book Group, Inc.
The Grand Central Publishing name and logo is a trademark of Hachette Book Group, Inc.

Printed in the United States of America

First Trade Printing: January 1999
First Mass Market Printing: March 2005

10 9 8 7 6 5 4

This book is dedicated to all the women who share their experiences with us and who teach us daily.

Acknowledgments

We would especially like to thank the many dedicated scientists, researchers, and clinicians whose work has contributed so greatly to this book, including David Zava, Ph.D., Christiane Northrup, M.D., Robert Gottesman, M.D., Marcus Laux, N.D., Mark Hochwender, and Raymond Peat, Ph.D. The courageous and pioneering research of Ercole Cavalieri, M.D., Kent Hermsmeyer, Ph.D., William Hrushesky, M.D., Peter Collins, M.D., Bent Formby, Ph.D., and T. S. Wiley is a major contribution to our understanding of the inner workings of hormones. Special thanks to Melissa Lowenstein for her research and writing assistance, to Tu Pham for her artwork, and to our editor Colleen Kapklein at Warner, who will be missed. Our individual personal thanks for their support and love go to Pat Lee, Liz Lee, Larry Johns, Elizabeth Renaghan, Mary Hopkins, Sri Gary Olsen, and Dennis Holtje.

Contents

Note from Dr. Lee   xiii

Note from Dr. Hanley   xvii

Part I: GETTING ACQUAINTED
     Life Cycles and Hormone Cycles   1

Chapter 1 Premenopause as a Life Cycle   3

Chapter 2 The Importance of Hormone Balance   23

Chapter 3 The Estrogens: Angels of Life, Angels
     of Death   48

Chapter 4 Progesterone and Progestins: The Great
     Protector and the Great Impostors   61

Chapter 5 How We Got into Xenohormone
     Hell—and How to Get Out   84

Part II: WHEN YOUR BODY TALKS, LISTEN
             *What's Causing Premenopause Syndrome
             Symptoms and How to Treat Them*   101

Chapter 6 How (and Why) to Keep Your Uterus
             and Save Your Cervix   103

Chapter 7 Cycles, Follicles, and Ovaries   125

Chapter 8 PMS: And When She Was Good She
             Was Very, Very Good, and When She
             Was Bad She Was Horrid   144

Chapter 9 Tired Adrenals Equals a Tired
             Woman   163

Chapter 10 Other Premenopause Syndrome
             Symptoms and Solutions   173

Chapter 11 The Dangers of Hormonal
             Contraceptives   219

Chapter 12 The Relationship of Hormones
             to Breast Cancer and Other
             Women's Cancers   226

Part III: THE PREMENOPAUSE BALANCE
             PROGRAM
             Practical Steps for Optimal Health   267

Chapter 13 Restoring and Maintaining
             Balance   269

Chapter 14 How Nutrition Affects Your
Hormone Balance 284

Chapter 15 How Exercise Affects Your
Hormone Balance 337

Chapter 16 How to Use Natural Progesterone 354

Chapter 17 How to Use Other Natural Hormones 372

Glossary 385

Resources 391

Recommended Reading 401

References 407

Bibliography 425

Index 427

About the Authors 439

Note from Dr. Lee

— ❦ —

When I self-published my book for doctors on the use of natural progesterone in 1993, little did I know, as I shipped books out of my garage, that my desire to spread the word about natural hormone balance would evolve into a full-time calling. Since then, my second book, *What Your Doctor May* Not *Tell You about Menopause*, has sold over half a million copies, and I have given hundreds of talks to tens of thousands of people all over the world. At least half a dozen other books have been published on the subject of using natural hormones, and the business of selling natural progesterone creams has grown from three companies to dozens.

Other more subtle but important changes have also taken place. The term *estrogen dominance*, which I coined in my first book, has entered mainstream medicine, and I've also noticed that the majority of researchers and doctors have now begun to make the key distinction between the synthetic progestins, such as Provera, and progesterone.

Some things haven't changed. The media continue to obediently parrot drug company press releases about biased, sloppy hormone studies without bothering to look at the studies with a critical eye. (Drug companies will spend $3 billion on advertising this year, so it's easy to see how they would exert a lot of control over the media.) Some of the claims made are ridiculous. For example, when all the media coverage about estrogen's beneficial effects on Alzheimer's disease began, it was based on one study with twelve women for a few months.

As I have traveled around the world giving talks, I've noticed that the women in the audience aren't all of menopausal age; many are younger and looking for answers to health problems they intuitively know are hormonal in nature. This book is for them. Premenopause syndrome, as I have come to call it, is widespread among women as much as twenty years before menopause. I have also discovered that premenopause syndrome predisposes a woman to have more problems during and after menopause, so it's well worth learning how to bring the body back into balance as soon as symptoms appear.

As a doctor in family practice for thirty years, I learned early on that my patients' problems had as much to do with their emotional well-being as their physical well-being, and that is perhaps even more true as it applies to women suffering from premenopause syndrome. The prospect of aging is much more daunting for a woman than it is for a man, so those first signs of hormonal imbalance that a woman experiences can give rise to emotional issues that can make the physical problems worse. To add insult to injury, if a woman goes to a doctor who practices conventional medicine, the solutions she is offered are likely to fall into two categories: surgery or drugs. Both are likely to make her problems worse instead of better.

For this new book, Virginia Hopkins and I invited Jesse Hanley, M.D., to add her expertise on healing the emotional and spiritual aspects of premenopause syndrome, as well as the use of nutritional supplements and herbs. Dr. Hanley's fifteen years of medical practice, including an active current practice in family medicine with an emphasis on women's health, will bring empathy and understanding to our readers. Every day she sees women who have premenopause syndrome, and she has become widely known for her unique ability to work in partnership with women to bring them back to health.

I encourage women reading this book to also read *What Your Doctor May* Not *Tell You about Menopause.* Even if you are twenty years away from menopause, it is an excellent source of information on how hormones, environmental toxins, nutrition, and exercise affect your health. It challenges much of the current information you'll find in the media on hormones, and delves into how the politics of selling drugs affects your health.

This new book gives women in their premenopausal years the knowledge, and thus the power, to stay healthy and whole, and to create the health program that works best for them.

Note from Dr. Hanley

———————— ❦ ————————

*C*reating a positive premenopause is extremely important to you and to the next generation of women. As I'm sure you yourself have experienced, girls in this culture are challenged on every level to maintain their sense of themselves and their health. They're entering puberty earlier and having sex sooner, with none of the maturity needed to meet the risks and responsibilities that go with it. They are forced to grow up sooner both because they are exposed to the adult world through the media, and because the sea of environmental estrogens we are living in is forcing their bodies into early puberty.

One of the greatest gifts of my life as a doctor is to help prepare young women to be healthy and whole adults and to help prepare premenopausal women to be healthy, content menopausal women. Because I'm a family doctor, I get to grow up and mature with them. I get to talk with girls about their first periods and give them a new way of understanding that their menstrual blood is sacred and not something to be ashamed of. I get to tell premenopausal women that when they are premenstrual they become more sensitive, even psychic—they become the oracles of the tribe. In our culture this heightened sensitivity has been called crazy and emotional, but I teach women that we must relearn to cherish, value, and seek out women for their sensitive nature.

Those of you who are now or soon to be pre-menopausal have a unique historical opportunity to recreate the experience in a positive way both for yourself and for the women who follow you. You can use your power as mothers, workers, and consumers to create positive change in the world. You can stand up for what is going to sustain the earth for countless generations, for what is good in our culture, for the health and well-being of our food chain, for our tribe, for your families, and your selves.

Women in their thirties to fifties are getting their chance to bond and band together, and to come from a loving and inspiring place instead of a place of fear. We are not at risk of being burned at the stake for knowing how to heal our children or ourselves as we were in the Dark Ages, when we were called witches and only men were allowed to have any wisdom or power. We have a sacred duty to reshape the future for ourselves, our children, and our planet.

I liked to call the process of a woman moving from her premenopausal years into her menopausal years "wisening." When you're wisened, you're in a position to say, "My dears, now that I know I have options, and I can see there are twenty-five different ways to do this, to hell with that one." What we're able to do in those wisening years a twenty-one-year-old could not do, regardless of how savvy she is. A younger woman does not have the distance, the perspective, the bangs, the bruises, the experience, the emotions, and the objectivity that a forty-year-old has to evaluate, discriminate, and make decisions.

For women who dread the prospect of menopause, I can tell you from my own experiences that fifty is not the end of your life but rather a very powerful beginning where you have the opportunity to rebirth your selves. You have been birthed by another, you may have birthed others, and now you get to birth your self. You will find that it is a sacred honor and privilege to get to know yourself and to stand as a woman of power and wisdom. My hope is that this book will help you bring great good health, inner strength, and emotional balance to your wisening years.

Part I

GETTING ACQUAINTED

Life Cycles and Hormone Cycles

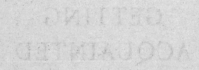

Chapter 1

❧

Premenopause as a Life Cycle

You're only in your mid-thirties and you absolutely do not want to hear the word "menopause" applied to you, even if it is "pre" menopause. You're not there yet. You're still young, you haven't even had kids yet for heaven's sake, or your kids aren't even out of grade school. And yet you know something in your body isn't quite right. You haven't changed your eating or exercise habits, but you're gaining weight. Your breasts are sore and lumpy, especially premenstrually, and you've started to have irregular periods. Maybe you've lost some of your sex drive or your skin is dry or isn't as smooth as it used to be. You used to think of yourself as very even-tempered, but lately you're irritable and snappish, and you can't seem to get out of bed in the morning. You have friends your age who are struggling with infertility, uterine fibroids, and premenstrual syndrome (PMS) when they've never had it before.

What's going on? It's premenopause syndrome, which is not a natural or inevitable part of life but rather one created by our culture, lifestyles, and environment.

Premenopause syndrome is a phenomenon that all women know about, but very few have a name for. Some fifty million women are going through premenopause right now, and most of them have experienced some form of this syndrome, which is a collection of symptoms experienced by women for ten to twenty years before menopause.

We call this *pre*-menopause rather than using the medical term *peri*menopause, because premenopause syndrome can begin as early as the mid-thirties whereas perimenopause technically means "right around menopause," meaning the year or two before, during, and after menstrual cycles end.

If you're a woman between the ages of thirty and fifty, you know a woman, maybe yourself, who has fibroids, tender or lumpy breasts, endometriosis, PMS, difficulty conceiving or carrying a pregnancy to term, sudden weight gain, fatigue, irritability and depression, foggy thinking, memory loss, migraine headaches, very heavy or light periods, bleeding between periods, or cold hands and feet. These symptoms are part of premenopause for a majority of today's women, and are the result of hormone imbalances, most of them caused by an excess of the hormone estrogen and a deficiency of the hormone progesterone. As you'll discover as you read on, natural progesterone is essential for maintaining hormone balance, and yet it has been largely overlooked by conventional medicine because of medical politics and pharmaceutical company profits.

However, premenopause symptoms are not just about biochemistry. They are also about women who are out of touch with the cycles and rhythms of their bodies, their feelings, and their souls. These are women who struggle to balance families and work, women who forget to take care of themselves, and women who aren't getting the help they need from their health maintenance organization (HMO).

There was a time when a woman's mother, grandmother, and aunts would quietly let her know what to expect during each phase of her life and help her through the rough patches with herbs and homespun, time-tested wisdom. These days the medical profession has taken over the role of a woman's extended family, but sadly, the advice they have to give out has more to do with dispensing drugs and scheduling surgery than with solutions that are healing—or that even work!

When women have premenopausal symptoms, estrogen is commonly prescribed. When that causes irregular bleeding or cervical dysplasia, or doesn't help their symptoms, their doctors often then resort to surgically induced menopause in the form of a hysterectomy, or they try personality-altering drugs such as Prozac and Zoloft to medicate them until they get through this particular phase of their lives. Or they are given more synthetic hormones—and the wrong hormones at that. None of these approaches really improves the quality of a woman's life, and they all have grave potential to cause illness and even to be life-threatening. In spite of what a conventional doctor will tell you, you *can* do something about the symptoms of premenopause besides antidepressant drugs, synthetic hormones, and surgery. We're not trying to say you will never have any symptoms as your hormones wind down or that you can live forever or that your skin will stay smooth and unwrinkled until you're ninety. But you definitely do not have to suffer from lumpy breasts, fibroids, and many of the other symptoms that show up anywhere from five to twenty years before menopause.

✤ LOOKING FORWARD TO MENOPAUSE

One of the reasons that premenopausal women don't want to talk about menopause is that they dread this hallmark of aging. This attitude is sad and contributes heavily to the emotional causes of premenopause symptoms. This attitude is particularly true of the many women who have postponed having children and who wonder if they're going to be able to have children before their biological alarm clock goes off.

Women have been taught in countless ways that their value lies in their ability to be sexually attractive to and unconditionally supportive of men, as well as being unselfishly maternal and unconditionally loving of their children. While these are truly positive feminine traits, they are also one-sided. A woman who has only developed these traits without developing her sense of self will be terrified at the prospect of aging. When her children have left the house, her breasts are sagging, and her skin is wrinkling, what does she have left?

Women who only develop this side of themselves also tend not to have good boundaries. They have spent so many years making themselves totally and selflessly available to their husbands and children that they don't know where their families end and they begin. They have trouble saying no and would be hard pressed to tell you when they last had an hour to themselves—or what they'd most like to do with an hour if they had one. It's no wonder that the process of becoming a more individualized and free woman can be a frightening one. These women are craving self-definition: Who am I? What's important to me? What really matters? What am I teaching my kids? What values do I stand for in my work? What are my personal creative gifts? They have to relearn their right to say, "No, I won't do that"; "No, I don't have time"; and "No, I'm not available right now."

Once a woman passes over the threshold of menopause and begins to redefine herself, she has the potential to discover the richest time of her life. She can look back on the energy and enthusiasm of youth as a thrilling and exciting time. Childbirth and parenting were magical and rewarding. A career was creative and empowering. Now her first fifty years of life are digested and integrated into wisdom and freedom. If you talk to menopausal women you will find that once a woman comes across the fifty threshold and gets a year or two over it, very few would go back for anything other than a tight butt and fewer wrinkles. Menopause was once called the "dangerous age" because so many women begin speaking their minds at that time of life. What the world needs more than anything is for a woman to have the courage to speak her mind.

Menopause is a life cycle to be respected and looked forward to. In the future, menopausal women will once again be cherished and appreciated for the experience they bring to the rest of us and looked upon as role models by younger women for their sense of individuality.

✤ CREATING A POSITIVE PREMENOPAUSE CYCLE

Before puberty, you had the freedom of living without hormonal cycles and the relatively steady physical and emotional balance of that freedom. During puberty, you rode the ups and downs of a body getting used to the surges of sex hormones and menstrual cycles as well as the growth of pubic hair, breasts, and a libido. In your twenties and early thirties, if you were lucky, you experienced a remarkable period of high energy, clear thinking and all the excitement, privileges, and challenges of being an adult and building your adult life. This is also a time when your hormones reach their maximum hum. There's a rhythm working that is so genetically empowered that it's harder for all the spiritual, psychological, and environmental challenges you have to knock it off balance.

Sometime between your mid-thirties and mid-forties this strong, vibrant cycle becomes more easily influenced by outside factors and lifestyle choices. You notice things are changing again. Your periods aren't as regular as they once were, and your breasts get painfully lumpy when you're premenstrual. Sometimes your periods are heavier or lighter than usual. You're at least a little moodier than you used to be, and you tire more easily. You don't recover as quickly from a long trip or a late night out. You need more sleep, or you aren't sleeping as well. You strain your muscles more easily when you exercise and find yourself grunting a little when you stand up. If you eat poorly or miss a meal, you notice it. Those onion rings you used to scarf down without consequences now give you heartburn, and just one too many glasses of wine gives you a headache. You aren't quite the sexual tigress you used to be, and sometimes you notice you're not as lubricated during intercourse. You used to have mild PMS, but now it's distracting and unpleasant. Even though your diet and exercise are the same, you've gained a little weight, and no matter what you do it doesn't come off and stay off. You're sprouting more than a few gray hairs, and if you're over forty, chances are good that you need reading glasses, at least for the fine print.

These are the signs of a midcycle of life when everything is changing again. It's not as short, intense, and dramatic as puberty for most women, but once again your hormones are fluctuating up and down, with a gradual and overall direction of winding down (see figure 1.1).

The premenopause life cycle is an extremely potent and empowering time of life. A balanced premenopausal

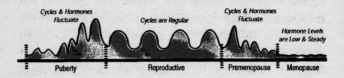

Figure 1.1. Hormones Across Your Life Span

woman is confident, knows herself, and has enough experience to be moving around in the world with self-assurance. She realizes that Prince Charming is not going to gallop up and rescue her, so she is no longer looking outside of herself for security. She has achieved a level of competence in the home and the workplace, as well as familiarity with her own strengths and weaknesses. One of the keys to a healthy premenopause cycle is to make it not just okay but wonderful to be moving into a time of life when we're becoming less physically powerful but more emotionally and spiritually powerful.

Anne

Anne is a forty-four-year-old schoolteacher who went to her doctor a year ago complaining of weight gain, depression, and headaches. She had also been having irregular periods for about six months. The depression and headaches were very difficult for her to cope with while teaching a class of energetic junior high schoolers. On many occasions she had found herself uncharacteristically snapping at her students or on the verge of tears.

She and her husband didn't have any children, but they were avid weekend hikers and loved to travel the world to beautiful hiking spots. Anne's weight gain had made it difficult for her to keep up on the hikes, and her depression made it hard just to get out of bed on weekends. Anne was nearly thirty pounds overweight, and her face was flushed, as if she had a permanent blush.

When Anne went to her HMO's doctor, he told her she was going into menopause, and gave her a prescription for Premarin, a synthetic estrogen and Provera, a synthetic progesterone. She dutifully took them, and for about two weeks she felt better. Then her symptoms started to become worse than before she had begun taking the synthetic hormones, and every time she took the Provera in the middle of her cycle her depression became dramatically worse. When she called her doctor to tell him, he called in a stronger dose of estrogen to the pharmacy, which Anne began taking. Within two weeks of the new regimen she had gained six pounds and was almost constantly weepy. She was calling in sick to work because her headaches had become so severe.

After six months of enduring these symptoms and on the verge of losing her job, Anne returned to her doctor for a pap smear and it came back positive for cervical dysplasia, a potentially precancerous condition. He told her that although they could take a wait-and-see approach for six months, he recommended a hysterectomy. He promised her that after the hysterectomy, all her symptoms would disappear and she would be a much happier woman.

At this point Anne went to see Dr. Hanley, weeping through most of the appointment. She confessed that she thought some of her depression was caused by the realization that at this late stage of her life she wanted a child, even though her husband was adamantly against it, to the point of not wanting to have sex for fear of pregnancy. Anne said with a sad laugh that her sex drive had disappeared since she had started taking the synthetic hormones, so she didn't really mind that her husband didn't want to have sex.

Dr. Hanley suggested to Anne that she keep a daily journal of her feelings, including her feelings about not having a baby. She explained that while Anne's symptoms were no doubt partly related to her conflict over having a baby, the severity of her headaches, depression, and weight gain, as well as her cervical dysplasia, had probably been caused by the high doses of estrogen she had been taking, as well as the synthetic progestins. Dr. Hanley did hormone tests, which revealed that Anne's level of follicle-stimulating hormone (FSH) was still normal, but her estrogen level was way too high, an indication that she was not in menopause yet. She suggested that they gradually ease her off the synthetic hormones, replacing them with natural progesterone. Dr. Hanley asked Anne to take the vitamin folic acid along with sublingual vitamin B12 and vitamin A to help heal the cervical dysplasia. She was asked to return in eight weeks for another pap smear.

Dr. Hanley also asked Anne to take up a gentle but regular weight-lifting program at the gym to bring her metabolism back to normal and help her reduce weight. Anne added twenty minutes on the treadmill and said the workout immediately picked up her energy and she felt more hopeful and cheerful.

Six months later, Anne had lost twenty pounds, and her last pap smear came back normal. She said that within days of beginning on the natural progesterone it felt as if her body was giving a huge sigh of relief, and her symptoms began to get better. She was bubbling over with energy and enthusiasm for a hike in the Peruvian Andes she and her husband were going on in a few weeks. She still felt sad about not having a child, but after many months of writing in her journal, she decided that her marriage was more important.

❧ LEARNING TO CREATE BALANCE

It's easy to believe that you're immortal up to your mid-thirties or mid-forties, when the evidence is piling on that aging is in process. But if you take care of yourself now, your aging process will happen later in life and will be more gradual and less debilitating. If you do your best to maintain your physical, mental, and emotional balance through the midcycle of your life, aging will be more graceful and less painful. You'll notice that balance is a key concept in this book and is the foundation of our Premenopause Balance Program.

Marie

Marie is a very thin, attractive thirty-nine-year-old attorney with a six-figure income and a corporate career that consumes her life. She lives in a big city in a fancy condo with a doorman and spectacular views of the city, drives an expensive car, and wears nothing but the finest clothes. She works out at the gym five mornings a week to maintain her trim figure and is careful about the foods she eats. She doesn't walk through the hallways of her office—she zooms. Marie is in perpetual motion all day and sometimes into the evening when she is dining with clients or traveling. In the car she is on her cell phone, and on airplanes the portable computer comes out. No moment is wasted.

When Marie was in her twenties, she assumed that she would eventually marry and have children, but that plan faded. She didn't even have plants or pets that would interfere with her busy travel schedule, and she decided that she didn't have time for children. She'd like to be married, she thinks, and she's usually dating a corporate executive or two, but in the past few years none of her relationships have lasted more than six months.

About a year before Marie went to see Dr. Hanley she ended up in a gynecologist's office because of severe, debilitating cramps in the middle of her menstrual cycle and spotty bleeding throughout her cycle. She was also waking up in the middle of the night drenched in sweat, which she was afraid might be a symptom of cancer. After a long series of tests, her gynecologist recommended a minor exploratory surgery to rule out cancer. Nothing terrified Marie more than surgery except the threat of cancer, which ran in her family, so she very reluctantly agreed to it. Her doctor found that she didn't have cancer, she had cysts on her ovaries. Some of them, the doctor reported, even had hair growing on them, and the very thought of that horrified Marie. The doctor removed one ovary that he judged irreparably damaged.

After the surgery Marie's doctor told her that if she continued to have problems she could have a hysterectomy and she could then be put on hormone replacement therapy (HRT). The prospect of major surgery, and of being on HRT, was unthinkable to Marie. A year later, when her symptoms had been recurring for a few months, she made an appointment with Dr. Hanley, hoping for an alternative to surgery and synthetic hormones. She was once again having heavy cramps, irregular bleeding, and night sweats, and she was also experiencing vaginal dryness and pain during intercourse.

The first thing she said to Dr. Hanley after describing her symptoms was, "I know that these are symptoms of menopause, but I'm not even forty yet. How can I be in menopause—I'm not ready for that!"

When Dr. Hanley asked about her lifestyle, Marie admitted that she knew she drank too much coffee, and she knew that caused her stomach pain and heartburn. "But," she said, "I can't seem to get going in the morning without it, and every time I try to quit I get terrible headaches." She added that in the afternoons she drank diet sodas containing caffeine and that in the evenings she might tend to have a glass or two more wine than is good for her. "But I need it to unwind and get to sleep," she explained.

Dr. Hanley explained to Marie that from the Chinese medicine point of view she was driving her male side very hard and neglecting her female side and that her first step in healing was going to be to bring these two parts of her self into balance. The driving, successful corporate executive who zoomed about and never paused was thriving at the expense of her more reflective, nurturing feminine side.

Not only were her malfunctioning ovaries symbolic of suppressing her feminine side, but also she probably wasn't making much in the way of hormones. Her remaining ovary was probably suppressed and her adrenal glands probably exhausted. That was causing the night sweats and hot flashes, a sign of low estrogen. Dr. Hanley measured Marie's hormones and found that they were very low. Marie was very resistant to the idea of taking any kind of hormones, even natural hormones in a cream, but she agreed to make some dramatic lifestyle changes to heal her body and bring herself back into balance and to take some herbs to help balance her hormones and support her adrenal glands.

When Marie returned a few weeks later, she told Dr. Hanley that after her first visit she had a dream that the hairy cyst on her ovary was a testicle and that graphic vision had been a great inspiration to make the necessary changes in her life to create more balance!

The first thing Marie did was announce to her partners at the office that she was cutting her client load in half and hiring a young attorney to travel in her place. She started taking painting classes and fulfilled a lifetime dream of spending a month in Paris in the spring, painting. When she returned, she bought a weekend house in the country, where she planned to paint, garden, and take long walks on the beach.

Marie also made smaller but equally important changes. She taught herself to walk slowly through the hallways of her office instead of zooming, she listened to soothing music in the car instead of making phone calls, and when she did have to travel she brought along a good novel instead of working on her portable computer. She cut down her time at the gym to three days a week and allowed herself to gain a little weight. With the help of a special herbal and nutritional supplement regimen prescribed by Dr. Hanley, she switched from coffee to herbal tea, stopped drinking sodas, and kept her wine consumption to a glass with dinner.

A year after her first visit with Dr. Hanley, Marie reported that her symptoms were 90 percent gone and that she felt she could live with the ten percent that were left. She had met a wonderful man, an artist himself, at her weekend home, and she'd been dating him for months to the exclusion of anyone else. She said she realized that it was her slower, more contemplative and creative lifestyle that had created the space for a relationship.

✤ SELFISHNESS

Women tend to be unclear that selfishness can actually be a good thing. Most women are taught as young girls that if they ever do or want anything for themselves they are selfish. They are trained from early on that their role in life is to be there for everyone else. Now it's time that women take back responsibility for their bodies, their emotional lives, their children, and their environment. That's selfishness with a capital *S*. Imagine how quickly pesticide-tainted food would disappear if women with families refused to buy anything but organic food. Imagine how quickly mainstream medicine would shift from a drugs-and-surgery to a prevention-and-healing mode if premenopausal women walked out on doctors who weren't helping them.

If a child has a chronic runny nose and ear infections it is likely caused by a food allergy inherited from the parent. If the mother is not willing to give up milk products to find out if a food allergy exists, how does she expect the child to give them up? If the mother is not doing what's good for her, how is the child going to learn to do what's best for him- or herself? Parents who are sexually abusive to each other will have children who grow up to be sexually abused. A parent who is exhausted and overwhelmed all the time will raise children who abuse themselves in the same way. We all learn by example. You can't help your children if you won't help yourselves.

One of the ways of being selfish in a good way is to

trust your heart and your intuition to be strong enough to insist on what you know, and to act on it.

Susan

Susan is thirty-five years old and has been married to an electrician for nine years with whom she has a three-year-old son named Adam. Susan works part-time for the phone company to help ends meet, since her husband's business always seems to be struggling, but the cost of day care means at the end of the day she has barely made minimum wage. Susan and her husband want another child and have been trying to get pregnant for a year.

Susan came to Dr. Hanley complaining of fatigue, heavy periods, and puzzlement over her inability to get pregnant, since it had happened so quickly with Adam. She looked pale and drawn, with dark circles under her eyes. She was about twenty pounds overweight, with most of it in her stomach and hips.

When Dr. Hanley gave Susan a vaginal exam, she found a fibroid the size of a golf ball on her uterus, which explained the heavy periods and perhaps difficulty in conceiving. Many doctors would have immediately scheduled Susan for surgery to remove the fibroid, and some even would have advised her that she would be unable to have another baby and recommended a hysterectomy.

Dr. Hanley sat down and had a talk with Susan after the exam. As they examined her life, Susan realized that she was ambivalent about having another baby when they really couldn't afford it, and she already seemed to be exhausted all the time. Another baby seemed inconceivable, and so it was!

Susan decided that what she needed first was to take care of herself, and once she gave herself permission to do that, she knew exactly what she needed. Adam still frequently woke up at night, and she was the one to go to him, so she was often sleep deprived. Susan decided she'd begin taking care of herself by asking her husband to spend Sunday mornings with Adam so she could sleep in. One morning a week of sleeping in sounded like heaven to her. She also resolved to take more long, hot bubble baths before bed and to be less of a perfectionist about how clean the house was. She looked considerably brighter after deciding to take just those three steps.

Dr. Hanley also recommended that Susan drink more water, eat more vegetables, and take a multivitamin. Then she explained that Susan was probably low on progesterone and suggested a series of tests done throughout the month to measure her hormone levels. In the meantime, she started her on a good multivitamin and some Chinese herbs.

Susan's test results did show that she was low on progesterone and also dehydroepiandrosterone (DHEA), so Dr. Hanley prescribed a regimen of a natural progesterone cream and a low dose of DHEA for three months.

Within three months Susan's energy was up, though not all the way. Her periods were normal, and her fibroid was clearly shrinking. Her husband had decided to go into partnership with another electrician, and they had postponed trying to get pregnant until they were more economically stable so that Susan could stop working when the new baby came.

Six months later, Susan was alive with energy, her eyes sparkled, her periods were normal, and her fibroid was undetectable. Within a year, she was pregnant.

In this chapter you have read about three very different women, but all with the same problem—premenopause syndrome. Their personalities, lifestyles, genetic makeups, and bodies are very different, but their health and emotional problems arise out of the same cycle of life, the premenopause cycle. A combination of an aging body, an imbalanced lifestyle, and a unique mix of physical predispositions set up each woman to have her particular problems.

It is our hope that you will use this book as a resource for creating a healthy, balanced premenopause cycle for yourself. We're going to show you how and why your body isn't working the way it used to and give you very practical, down-to-earth solutions that really work. But we're not offering any magic pills here. Up until our late twenties or early thirties we can get away with a lot when it comes to lifestyle choices. We can party into the wee hours, drink too much alcohol, and manage to show up functional for work the next day; we can subsist largely on a diet of soft drinks, French fries, and candy bars and still be reasonably healthy. But as we get older, we can get away with less and less, and by the time we're in our forties, if we have been careless with our bodies, we've created chronic health problems that resist conventional treatments. With the information and resources provided in this book, you can make the premenopause cycle of your life a healthy, energetic, and deeply rewarding one.

When you reach menopause, you'll be back to having lower and more stable hormone levels, with all the steadiness that goes with it, but this time you'll be in an adult body and will experience tremendous freedom and creativity. Most women love it once they get there. And these days, with the help of natural hormones and a healthy lifestyle, you can maintain your health and your sexuality like never before and fully enjoy the wisdom and privileges of growing older.

Since *What Your Doctor May Not Tell You about Menopause* was written, the amount of new research and clinical information we have about premenopause syndrome has grown exponentially. We know much more about what happens to a woman's biochemistry as she ages, and so much more about what drives the hormone-related cancers that begin to strike at that age, that we want to share what we know with you. We have startling new revelations to share, and can now state with authority what was only theorized or hinted at a few years ago.

If you're suffering from premenopause syndrome, there are very specific causes and very specific solutions. Every woman's combination of genetics, personality, biochemistry, and lifestyle is different, so every woman's health solutions will be unique to her. Consider this book a road map. You can become acquainted with what it has to offer and then choose your own personal path to health. Bon voyage!

Chapter 2

The Importance of Hormone Balance

Denise was thirty-six when her gynecologist told her that the only way he could treat her severe endometriosis was to put her on birth control pills containing a synthetic progestin. She had been on birth control pills in her early twenties and they had made her feel tired and cranky, so she was reluctant to try them again. She had also done her homework and knew that birth control pills increased her risk of having a stroke, even at her young age. But Denise was so tired of having severe cramps and pain before and during her periods that she was ready to do just about anything to relieve the problem. In fact, in the months before she saw her doctor, she had been forced to take nearly a week off from work because of the pain. She worked in a highly competitive corporate environment, and taking that much time off from work was frowned upon. She felt her job was in jeopardy.

Denise began taking a progestin-only birth control pill at the beginning of her next cycle, and noticed that she did have less pain and cramping during her next cycle. By the second month she had even less pain, but she also noticed that the fine, downy hair on her face had grown thicker. By the third month her symptoms had been reduced by at least half, but she had grown a couple of thick, black hairs around her chin, she was losing some hair at her temples, and the hair on her arms was thicker. She also noticed that she was much more impatient and irritable with her husband, and she experienced surges of anger that she had never felt before.

The imbalance of estrogen that stimulated the growth of the endometrial tissue in Denise's body and caused her pain had been somewhat balanced or opposed by the birth control pills she was given, but she was also suffering from the side effects of taking a progestin that had the qualities of a male hormone, or androgen, as well as some of the qualities of progesterone. Rather than achieving balance, she had traded one set of symptoms for another. The birth control pills Denise had been given were not truly progesterone, and not truly any single male hormone, but had the qualities of both. No wonder her body was confused.

Taking one of the strange, not-found-in-nature synthetic hormones created by the drug companies is one of the best and quickest ways to confuse your body and throw it into a state of imbalance. These drugs are created not because they work better than natural hormones but rather because they can be patented, and patent drugs have a much higher price tag than natural substances. Later in the book we'll explain in detail how Denise could have relieved her symptoms without creating new problems. In this chapter we'll look more closely at the concept of hormone balance at the molecular level so you'll have a better understanding of how it works in your own body and how even small changes in hormone balance can have dramatic effects on you.

❧ CONDUCTING YOUR HORMONE SYMPHONY

The function of your hormones is determined first and foremost by their specific molecular configuration, just as specific keys work in specific locks. And just as changing one small groove can make a key not fit in a lock, extremely small changes in molecular configuration can change how a hormone works.

The steroid hormones are very similar, but their effects are quite different. When you look at molecular diagrams of the steroid hormones—pregnenolone, progesterone, androstenedione, the estrogens, testosterone, DHEA, and the cortisols—they look almost exactly alike, with just one or two seemingly small differences (see figure 2.1). And yet those slight differences—a hydrogen atom here, a carbon atom there—make the difference between a man and a woman, pregnancy and infertility, fatigue and energy, premenopause symptoms and good health.

The coordinated movement of the manufacture and dispersal of hormones in a woman's body is like an orchestra, where all the instruments need to play together to achieve balance and harmony. It doesn't take much to throw the hormonal symphony into chaos. If the estrogen is too loud, the progesterone can't be heard. If cortisol is too high, it drowns out the progesterone and DHEA. If pregnenolone is low, all of the other hormones may miss their cues and drop notes.

The steroid hormones are made from cholesterol in the adrenal glands and ovaries of women, and there is mounting evidence that some are manufactured elsewhere in the body. For example, we know that estrogen can be manufactured by fat cells, and there's good evidence that progesterone is manufactured in the Schwann's cells that make up the myelin sheath that protects nerve cells.

The steroid hormones affect all parts of the body, including the brain, bones, circulation, digestion, liver, kidneys, nerves, muscles, reproductive organs, and the immune system. They have a powerful effect on your body's ability to resist disease, especially cancer, heart disease, respiratory diseases, arthritis, osteoporosis, brain diseases, and circulatory diseases.

The steroid hormones are intimately related to each other, each one being made from another or turned back into another depending on the needs of the body. For example, from progesterone your body can make DHEA, cor-

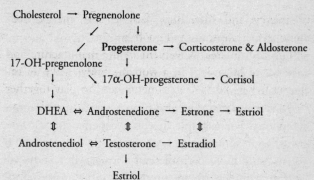

Figure 2.1. Hormone Pathways
Basic steroid hormone pathways in the ovary. Each arrow in the pathway represents the work of a specific enzyme and indicates the direction of the action. Only in a few instances is an action reversible, as indicated by the double arrows.

tisol, and estriol. Androstenedione can be transformed into testosterone and estrone, and testosterone can be made into estriol, estradiol, and androstenedione. (See figure 2.1 for a visual look at these relationships.) With all these interrelationships possible, you can imagine that if one of these hormones is missing, or is present in the wrong amount, it would have a profound effect on your body.

But the hormones themselves are just part of the picture. It takes very specific combinations of vitamins, minerals, and enzymes to cause the transformation of one hormone into another and then help the cell carry out the hormone's message. If you are deficient in one of the important hormone-transforming substances such as vitamin B6 or magnesium, for example, that too can throw your hormones out of balance. Thyroid and insulin problems, toxins, bad food and environmental factors, medication, and liver function affect nutrient and hormone balance.

Your emotional state also plays a role in the hormone symphony. For example, if you're experiencing chronic stress, your adrenal glands are pumping out cortisol. If you're using more cortisol than normal, your body will have to compensate by producing more progesterone from which to make the cortisols. Cortisol also stimulates the production of cholesterol, the building block of all the steroid hormones. Cortisol competes with progesterone in bone, and yet they give opposite messages. Progesterone tells bone cells to build, while cortisol tells bone cells to stop building. Both chronic stress and the cortisol drugs taken in excess can contribute to osteoporosis. Chronic stress that creates a chronic demand for cortisol will eventually lead to adrenal exhaustion and symptoms similar to chronic fatigue.

Similarly, chronic stress and hormone imbalance disrupt the brain and disrupt its signals to the hormone-producing glands. Your balance of steroid hormones can in turn affect your emotional state. Testosterone in excess stimulates aggression and anger, whereas estrogen in excess stimulates passivity and oversensitivity. DHEA can stimulate a feeling of well-being, whereas progesterone promotes feelings of calmness. Estrogen, which excites brain cells, can cause mental confusion and agitation in excess, whereas an estrogen deficiency can cause depression. Many people report feeling more mentally alert when they use pregnenolone, and we have heard from hundreds of women that using a progesterone cream dramatically reduced their feelings of anxiety.

The brain is the master switch that regulates hormone levels. The specific areas of the brain that control hormone levels are the hypothalamus and pituitary gland. If they are damaged, adversely affected by a genetic glitch, given mixed or confused messages by the rest of the body, or simply wearing out due to the aging process, hormone levels can be affected. In women, a surge of luteinizing hormone (LH) is released by the brain to cause the release of the egg from the ovary. Dr. Hanley is seeing more and more women in her office who have very low levels of LH, a sign that the brain is not functioning properly in relationship to their hormones. Not surprisingly, she is seeing the same thing in men, who also release LH to stimulate the production of testosterone. Dr. Hanley estimates that the majority of the men she tests who are age thirty and older are below the normal range of LH levels. This means that in many cases of infertility, it's not that the testicle couldn't and it's not that the ovary wouldn't; rather it's that these male and female gonads aren't getting the message from the brain. We can theorize that both stress and environmental chemicals are disrupting the brain, but we won't know for sure until it is researched and tested.

❧ THE MYTH OF "NORMAL" HORMONE LEVELS IN PREMENOPAUSAL WOMEN

Amy is a forty-one-year-old electrical engineer who likes to make decisions based on hard numbers and facts. She was having some hot flashes and was inexplicably gaining weight. When she went to her doctor, he recommended that she have her hormone levels tested. He sent in a blood hormone test for her that was taken during the middle of her menstrual cycle. It came back showing that she had extremely low levels of all the hormones measured. In fact, her levels were so low that her doctor decided to retest her on the following month at the same time in her cycle. Those results came back normal except for her testosterone, which came back high. He tested her testosterone levels again and they came back normal. With such inconsistent results, Amy felt she didn't have reliable information with which to make a decision about how to balance her hormones, so her doctor suggested she try a saliva hormone level test. She did, and the results came back equally inconsistent.

When you are a premenopausal woman, it can be difficult or even impossible to accurately measure your hormone levels because they fluctuate so much, especially in the few years before menopause. You could measure your hormones three times in one day and get drastically different readings each time, and you could measure them three times in a week and get the same widely varying results. We'll go into more detail on hormone testing later in the book, but for now what is important to know is that if you get your hormones measured and they are above or below normal, it's not time to panic. The premenopause cycle of your life is a time when your hormones are fluctuating. Hormones levels can vary widely from woman to woman without being abnormal.

If you measure the hormones of a hundred women who are on the same cycle, even before premenopause symptoms appear, you will find a wide variation, as much as fourfold either way. To give you a contrast, body temperature range is very tight, 98.6 degrees Fahrenheit. Just a degree or two up or down can reliably indicate a problem. The pH or acid-base range is even tighter. Calcium and phosphorus ratios can vary but only by about 5 percent. There are a lot of tight ranges in the body, but hormone levels aren't one of them. That's why we encourage you to become familiar with your symptoms and use them as your primary guide as to which hormones are out of balance. Testing hormone levels can be useful for some women, but we don't want you to panic if they seem inconsistent or you are told they are "abnormal."

❧ HORMONES AS MESSENGERS

We've looked at hormone balance like a symphony, but you can also look at specific hormones as individual messengers. There are a multitude of factors that may affect message reception. Let's look at some of the issues that can intervene, using the analogy of a messenger in the time of knights attempting to deliver a message to the queen in her castle.

1. *The message may not reach the intended receptor.* The messenger may be killed by bandits, never reaching the queen. For hormones to work, they must pass into cells to reach receptors within. Altered conditions around the outside of the cell can alter the passage of the hormone. In the case of the pancreatic hormone insulin, for example, this is called insulin resistance, which leads to diabetes. The insulin is there, but it is unable to deliver its message to the cell.

2. *The queen may not be in the castle. (The receptors may not be in the target cell.)* The messenger may get to the castle, but the queen might be off visiting another country. Three princesses offer to take the message, but the messenger has been instructed to give his message only to the queen. For hormones to work, they must pass through the cell and then unite with pre-formed receptors within the cell. How cell receptors are formed is strongly influenced by your genetics. Genetic glitches may occur which create too many, too few, or no appropriate hormone receptors. When this happens the hormone has no effect.

   An extreme example of absent receptors that was reported in a medical journal documents a young man who lacked all estrogen receptors. One of the effects that estrogen has in both males and females is to give the message to the growth plates in bones to close sometime after puberty. This young man had normal estrogen levels, but since he had no receptors his bones never got the message to stop growing. At age twenty-nine, his bones continued to grow, resulting in abnormal leg and arm length, which eventually will seriously increase his risk of fracture.

Another example comes from breast cancer researcher Dr. David Zava, who recalls a woman with normal progesterone levels who lacked progesterone receptors in her cells (a rare genetic abnormality). She developed breast cancer in her early twenties and died of it shortly thereafter.

Another example is the progesterone receptor itself. In ovary and breast cells, estrogen stimulates the formation of progesterone receptors. Progesterone cannot deliver its message to these cells unless estrogen has prepared the way. Breast cancer cells will not show positivity for progesterone receptors unless they also have estrogen receptors. The converse is not true: Estrogen receptors do not require the presence of progesterone, although they seem to be sensitized when progestrone is given to a woman who has been deficient in progestrone.

3. *The queen (receptor) may be present but unavailable, being occupied with other messages.* The messenger gets into the castle, but finds that the queen is in a meeting with her ministers and isn't available to receive his message. Hormones with different messages may nevertheless occupy the same receptors. The hormones are then said to compete with each other for the receptor sites. This is the case of cortisol and progesterone. Their molecular structures are very similar and both can occupy and thus compete for the same receptors in osteoblasts, the bone-building cells in bone. The message

of progesterone to osteoblasts is to *stimulate* them to make a new bone whereas the message of glucocorticoids to osteoblasts is to *inhibit* them from making new bone. Thus, the former prevents osteoporosis whereas the latter can cause osteoporosis. In general, an excess of cortisol that blocks progesterone's action can cause a de facto progesterone deficiency.

Similarly, synthetic progesterone-like compounds (progestins) also can occupy osteoblast-progesterone receptors. Despite being more potent at other sites, progestins are less potent than progesterone in promoting new bone formation. Also, being foreign to the usual metabolic pathways through which hormones move, synthetic progestins are more tenacious in the occupancy of these receptors and thus inhibit the message of progesterone even at low dosages.

4. *The message may be miscommunicated to or by the queen. (Genetic factors may change the hormone message.)* The messenger delivers his message to the queen, but she doesn't have her glasses and misunderstands the message. She passes on incorrect information to her generals, who lose a battle because they were misinformed. When a hormone arrives in a cell and unites with its receptor, it is carried into the cell nucleus where it fits a specific gene site to create a certain chromosomal response leading to some change in the cell's actions. Genetic glitches in the hormone-stimulated gene will alter the expression of the hormone's message. Though the message was received,

the action it was meant to produce will not occur as it was intended.

5. *The messenger is delayed or blocked. (Lack of appropriate cofactors can interfere with the message.)* The messenger sets out on his journey, but his horse falls and breaks a leg, or a storm forces him to seek cover for days. Most actions of cells are mediated by enzymes, vitamins, minerals, and other nutrients. If the nutrients are not available, enzyme activity is impaired. The hormone message effectively turns on the enzyme production, but the enzyme can't do its work adequately because one of its cofactors is missing.

6. *The message may be inhibited.* The messenger sets out on his journey, but halfway there he is captured by a rival queen and held hostage. Just as the presence of vitamins and minerals is important for optimal response, the presence of inhibiting factors is equally important because they can block optimal response. Excessive iron interferes with enzymes throughout the body. In the disease hemochromatosis, which causes excess iron to build up in the body, the symptoms include painful joints, coronary heart disease, and an increased incidence of colon and liver cancer. Excess iron inhibits enzyme messages and blocks the action of other minerals in the body. Fluoride does the same thing: Just as it interferes with dental enamel formation, leading to dental fluorosis (discolorations on the teeth), it also causes increased bone calcification in which the new bone formed is of poorer quality, leading to increased risk of fracture later in life. The hor-

mones for bone building are operating normally but the expression of the bone formed under the influence of excessive calcium is altered by the presence of this toxic factor.

Nutritional imbalances and environmental toxins commonly inhibit hormonal messengers.

7. *The volume of the message may be turned down or up.* The messenger delivers his message verbally to the queen, but he yells so loudly that two princesses also hear the message and take action themselves. Or he speaks softly, but since the queen is hard of hearing she doesn't know he gave her a message and she takes no action. One of the most intriguing things about hormones is that their volume, or level, alters the effect of their messages. In cooking, the presence of a little salt may be pleasing to one's taste, but excessive salt ruins the taste. A light touch of one's hand may be pleasing to another, but a harder touch can be painful. A whispered "I love you" is much more pleasing than the same words shouted in your face.

Even though estrogen and progesterone generally have opposing effects in cells, estrogen enhances progesterone action by being necessary for receptor formation, and progesterone can enhance estrogen action by up-regulating estrogen receptor sensitivity. If a woman is deficient in progesterone for an extended period of time, the return of low-dose progesterone will temporarily enhance estrogen breast receptor sensitivity. This is why so many women experience breast tenderness when they first start using a progesterone cream. When progesterone levels rise back to normal levels, the breast effects of estrogen are opposed and the breast tenderness goes away. The initial "touch" of progesterone temporarily increases the sensitivity of breast estrogen receptors, whereas higher levels tune them down.

Dr. David Zava has observed that excess progesterone results in higher cortisol levels, which can cause increased water retention. He believes that this is the cause of breast swelling sometimes caused by long-term progesterone supplementation or high-dose progesterone.

With all of these possible effects on hormone messages, it's easy to understand how balancing hormones isn't just a matter of supplementing one hormone, or using a hormone level test and then trying to adjust your hormones accordingly. Supplemental hormones by the bucketful won't bring your body back into balance if you're chronically exposed to stress, toxins, or a poor diet, for example. To use the analogy above, you can send out all the messengers you want to the queen, but if a key bridge is out none of them will get there. That's why we will continually be stressing throughout this book that achieving hormone balance is also a matter of achieving balance in your life as a whole.

❖ NATURAL VERSUS SYNTHETIC HORMONES

Not too long ago Dr. Lee was confronted at a conference by the owner of a large herbal products company who claimed that Dr. Lee was incorrect in referring to the progesterone used in the creams as "natural" because it was manufactured, or synthesized, in a laboratory and that made it synthetic. This is a confusion in semantics that we hear frequently. In fact, progesterone is far more natural to your body than any plant because your body actually manufactures the identical substance. The progesterone manufactured in the laboratory has the identical molecular configuration of the progesterone that your body makes. It does not matter if the body makes the hormone or if a chemist makes it from a plant extract or from anything else. If it is the identical molecule, it is the identical hormone. The source of the progesterone is unimportant in this context.

We usually think of the word *synthetic* as meaning something that is produced artificially and is not found in nature, such as plastics or pharmaceutical drugs. For example, the "hormone" Provera is made from the same substances that natural progesterone is made from, but the molecular configuration of it is changed in the laboratory so that it is not identical to anything found in nature. But natural progesterone made in the laboratory is identical to that made in the human body. In other words, what makes a substance "synthetic" or "natural" in this context is whether it can be found in nature and whether it is natural to the human body.

The same distinctions apply to estrogens. The two types of estrogen in Premarin taken separately are natural (found in nature) and not synthetic, but not all of the estrogen in Pemarin is natural to humans. About half of it is human estrogen, and about half is horse estrogen— a molecule not found in the human body. It's ironic that the manufacturer of Premarin has tried to advertise it as a natural product. Since about half of the estrogen in Premarin is estrone, which is natural to humans, and the other half consists of a different estrogen that is natural only to horses and is extracted from pregnant horse urine, it is natural, strictly speaking, only if you are half horse and half human! It's unfortunate that so much estrogen research has been done with Premarin, because we don't have a truly accurate knowledge base of the effects of human estrogen versus horse estrogen. In addition, recent research has shown that the "horse urine" part of Premarin contains over 100 active ingredients, including a measurable amount of progesterone. These revelations muddy the waters of estrogen research even more.

Natural estrogens synthesized from fats extracted from wild yams or soybeans that are identical to those made by the human body are easily available by prescription in the form of creams, tablets, and patches. These are estrone, estradiol, and estriol. There is no reason to take horse estrogen.

Plants do not make human hormones, but some plants make compounds that have some hormonal effect.

These, in their natural form, are called phytohormones (plant-based hormones). Although they are not the same as our hormones, they may have some hormonal activity. We'll cover those in more detail shortly.

Some plants make substances that are quite similar to animal cholesterol or animal hormones, but they have no hormonal effect. Such compounds, called sterols, are easily chemically modified to become identical to human hormones. An example of this is the diosgenin that is extracted from wild yams and soybeans to make human hormones in the laboratory.

In 1938 Dr. Russell E. Marker discovered how to convert diosgenin from wild yams into progesterone (see figure 2.2). Because his product was identical to human progesterone, we call it "natural" progesterone, that is, natural to humans. It is *not* called "natural" because it was chemically derived from a plant compound.

Since Dr. Marker made his discovery sixty years ago, other steroid hormones have also been manufactured from diosgenin. The medicine digoxin is also derived from diosgenin.

The phytohormones found in herbs are natural in that they are manufactured by nature, but they aren't natural to your body. Phytoestrogens in particular can be useful because they behave like weak-acting estrogens and do occupy estrogen receptors so they can protect against excess estrogen coming from the environment or from within the body. In women who are estrogen deficient they can supply a modest estrogen effect.

The use of herbs as medicines is generally preferable to

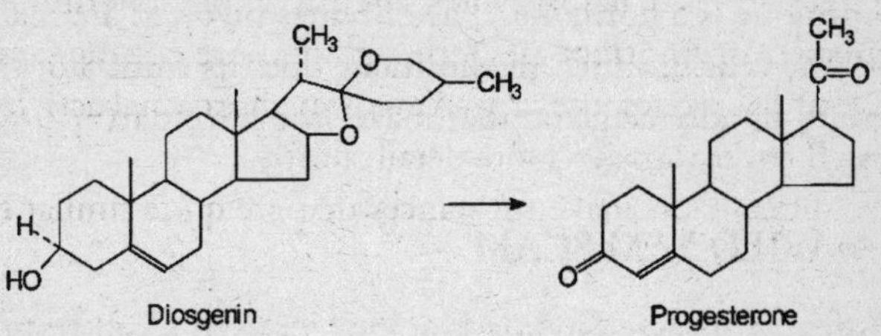

Figure 2.2. The Conversion of Diosgenin to Progesterone
The diosgenin molecule can be converted to a progesterone molecule in the laboratory, but not in the human body.

most prescription drugs because they tend to have a more gentle action and fewer side effects. The human body has spent millions of years evolving, and in that evolutionary process it has adapted elegantly to use the foods and medicines the earth provides in the form of plants. It is not surprising that we have learned to tolerate plant compounds pretty well. But there are many plants which contain compounds that are toxic to us—consider poisonous mushrooms and poison ivy for example. Therefore, just the fact that something comes from a plant does not guarantee it is good for us, even if it is manufactured by Mother Nature. If you are going to use herbs to balance your hormones, it is recommended that you consult with a qualified and experienced herbalist.

We have also heard people make claims that the pure progesterone made from wild yams or soybeans doesn't contain the enzymes necessary for the body to use it. This is an unfounded assumption not based on facts. A hormone is a hormone. The enzymes involved are made by the cells in which the hormone does its work, not the ovary or adrenal gland that makes the hormone.

❖ WILD YAM SCAM

A few years ago Virginia Hopkins received a call from a health food store in her area that sells progesterone creams. The manager of the store told her that a very angry woman in a wheelchair named Sally was in his store, and he wondered if he could put her on the phone to ask some questions. It seems that about ten months earlier Sally, a regular customer for years, had come into the store and told a clerk there that she had osteoporosis and had asked for anything that might help her. The clerk gave her a copy of *What Your Doctor May Not Tell You about Menopause* and a jar of "progesterone" cream. Sally went home and dutifully followed the directions in the book for using progesterone cream. Nine months later she broke her hip, and tests showed that her bone density had decreased. She was angry because the progesterone hadn't worked to stop her bone loss.

Virginia asked Sally many questions, from how much soda and meat she was consuming to how much weight-bearing exercise she had been getting to how her digestion was, but couldn't come up with an explanation of why the progesterone hadn't worked. Then she asked what kind of progesterone cream Sally was using. It turned out she wasn't using progesterone at all!

Sally had been using a product containing diosgenin

that was identified as "wild yam extract" on the jar. In the chemistry lab scientists can make progesterone from diosgenin. That does *not* mean that your body can make progesterone from diosgenin—or any other hormone for that matter. Those who sell diosgenin or diosgenin disguised as "extract of wild yam" or *Dioscorea* (the Latin name for the Mexican wild yam) in creams or capsules and claim that it has the same effect as progesterone are not speaking the truth. Sally is a tragic testimony to the inaccuracy of these types of misleading claims and products. Diosgenin is significantly less expensive than real progesterone, so greed, and not ignorance, may be the motivation for this practice.

Diosgenin is also added as an ingredient to many genuine progesterone creams, and it is usually identified as "dioscorea" or "wild yam extract." For the most part this is a marketing device designed to capitalize on the confusion between wild yam and progesterone. In most cases there's probably not enough diosgenin in these creams to have much of a physiologic effect. However, the truth is that we really don't know exactly what effect diosgenin has or even how well it is absorbed through the skin. We recommend that women who are pregnant or nursing use a cream that doesn't contain diosgenin, wild yam, or any other active ingredients whose effect is unknown.

To confuse matters even more, thirty years ago the original manufacturers of progesterone cream identified the progesterone in their product as "wild yam extract," to make the U.S. Food and Drug Administration (FDA) happy, and many manufacturers who followed copied them, so there are real progesterone creams out there that say "wild yam extract" on the label. Please make sure your source of progesterone cream is reliable. (See pages 391–396 for a list of creams that contain real progesterone according to an independent laboratory assay, in a high enough concentration to be useful.)

Similar claims are made for diosgenin and the hormone DHEA. Manufacturers put diosgenin or "wild yam " in a capsule and claim that it is DHEA. It's not! These companies have done many tests measuring hormone levels before and after taking these products, and the most they have done is raise cholesterol levels slightly.

There is no doubt that wild yams have some effect on the body. Many women report that they "perk up" when they use them. Biochemist David Zava, Ph.D., has studied wild yams in the laboratory and thinks they may support the adrenal glands in some way. A leaf of spinach contains over ten thousand different compounds. Mexican wild yams may contain that many or even more. The Chinese have used a type of wild yam for centuries to treat women's health problems, so there's a good chance that it has some benefit. We just don't know exactly what it is. What's important to know is that wild yam or diosgenin is not progesterone, it won't turn into progesterone in your body, and it does not have the benefits of progesterone. We recommend that if you want to try wild yam, get the Chinese type from a reputable source, and again, consult with a qualified herbalist.

✦ PHYTOHORMONES

Phytohormones refer to plant compounds with hormonal effects. Such compounds may convey estrogenic, androgenic, corticosteroid, or progesterone-like effects. The function of phytohormones is exceedingly complex and probably involves many other plant factors that, by synergy, enhance their hormonal effects. When ingested, plant compounds that convey hormone-like effects are absorbed and activate hormone receptors, usually with less effect than human hormones. In cases of hormone deficiency, they can provide hormone-like beneficial effects. Many herbs with hormonal effects are revered in medical folklore for benefits such as improved fertility, healthier babies, and relief of hormone-deficiency symptoms. Plants with well-known hormone-like actions include vitex (chaste tree), licorice, sarsaparilla, legumes such as soybeans, and the European mistletoe.

Women who eat a plant-based diet that is rich in a variety of fresh fruits and vegetables, and thus rich in phytohormones, are less likely to experience premenopausal or menopausal symptoms. Often, women who have mild symptoms of estrogen deficiency, such as hot flashes or vaginal dryness, can take herbs that are rich with phytoestrogens (compounds in plants with estrogenic effects), which will suffice. Thus, proper diet or herb supplements often makes prescription estrogen unnecessary. Throughout the book we will discuss the use of herbs to treat premenopausal symptoms.

❧ XENOHORMONES

Xenohormones, also called xenobiotics, are synthetic chemicals such as pesticides and plastics which exert hormonal influences on all living creatures, including insects, fish, reptiles, amphibians, birds, and mammals. They have become pervasive in our environment and are disrupting the reproductive abilities and hormonal balance of all living creatures, including humans. A majority of the xenohormones have estrogenic effects. Xenohormones are covered in detail in chapter 5.

❧ KNOW YOUR SYMPTOMS

Since premenopausal hormone levels can vary so dramatically even within the same day, it can be difficult to get an accurate reading of what's out of balance through a blood or a saliva test. A hormone that registers as very low one day could register very high the next day. The best approach is to become aware of your symptoms and look for patterns: Do they occur at the same time in your menstrual cycles, or at the same time every day? Do they happen after you've eaten certain foods or when you're under stress? Does exercise make things worse or better?

A daily journal can be invaluable in helping you detect patterns. You can even make yourself a chart of symptoms and check them off at the end of each day, or make notations on a calendar. Every woman's style is different. What's important is to track what's happening to you so that you can use the information to bring yourself into balance.

In the chapters that follow you'll learn about the two primary hormones that you need to keep in balance, relative to your body's overall needs and relative to each other within your body: estrogen and progesterone. We'll also take a brief look at the cortisols and the androgens, or male hormones, including DHEA, androstenedione, and testosterone.

Chapter 3

❖

The Estrogens: Angels of Life, Angels of Death

*B*ecause of their tremendous range of effects—from beneficial to harmful—the hormones known as estrogens were dubbed the "angels of life and the angels of death," by Dr. Ercole Cavalieri, a scientist who has spent the last three decades studying their effects. You'll learn more about his work in chapter 12.

Dr. Cavalieri's phrase is telling. An excess or a deficiency of estrogens can make a world of difference in a woman's outlook on life and in her overall health and well-being. For example, too much estrogen and you're likely to feel bloated and oversensitive, and have insomnia. Too little and you may feel mentally lethargic and depressed. Maintaining estrogen balance can be challenging for a premenopausal woman, but there are many ways to achieve balance, and we hope that by the time you finish this book you'll find it as easy as adjusting your diet slightly, getting some exercise, or rubbing on a dab of progesterone cream.

The word *estrogen* is not the name of any specific hormone; it is a class name for a large group of compounds with estrogenic properties. These include human estrogens, animal estrogens, synthetic estrogens, phytoestrogens, and xenoestrogens. The three major human estrogens are estradiol, estrone, and estriol.

A rise in estrogen at puberty is responsible for the development and maintenance of female sex organs and secondary sexual characteristics such as breasts and pubic hair as well as for maintenance of menstrual cycles and pregnancy. A primary role of estrogen is to control the growth and function of the uterus: Specifically, estrogens create the proliferative endometrium or the blood-rich lining of the uterus, preparing it for pregnancy.

Estrogen effects are also seen on the ovaries, cervix, fallopian tubes, vagina, external genitalia, and breasts. Vocal cord changes and fat deposition in the breasts and hip area are also attributable to estrogen. The emergence of estrogen at puberty stops the growth of long bones in both males and females. Just prior to puberty there is a spurt in height, but after puberty, when estrogen is higher, height does not increase.

As a general rule, estrogen stimulates cell growth. It is responsible for giving the female body the signals to build blood-rich tissue in the uterus in the first part of the menstrual cycle, and it is part of the hormonal signals

that stimulate the maturation of an egg-containing follicle in the ovary.

It is estrogen's tendency to stimulate cell growth that
makes its excess such a dangerous promoter of cancer.
This is why it is so important to use progesterone if you
have the symptoms of estrogen dominance (see the list
on pages 51–52) or if you are taking estrogen for hormone replacement. Progesterone gives your body the
ability to keep estrogen's cell growth properties in check.
We'll discuss estrogen and cancer in more detail in
chapter 12.

Estrogen's stimulatory effect on cell growth makes it
useful in wound healing. A recent study in the journal
Nature Medicine showed that wounds healed more slowly
in older women, though with less scarring. When they
were given estrogen, their healing time was improved.
Young female rats with their ovaries removed took significantly longer to heal wounds, but when topical estrogen was applied, the wound healed very quickly.

Excess estrogen tends to create deficiencies of zinc,
magnesium, and the B vitamins, all of which are important to the maintenance of hormone balance. Magnesium, sometimes called the antispasm nutrient, is
especially important in the prevention of heart attacks.

Estrogen dominance is a term coined by Dr. Lee in his
first book on natural progesterone. It describes a condition where a woman can have deficient, normal, or excessive estrogen but has little or no progesterone to
balance its effects in the body. Even a woman with low
estrogen levels can have estrogen-dominance symptoms

if she doesn't have any progesterone. The symptoms and conditions associated with estrogen dominance are:

Acceleration of the aging process

Allergy symptoms, including asthma, hives, rashes, sinus congestion

Autoimmune disorders such as lupus erythematosis and thyroiditis, and possibly Sjögren's disease

Breast cancer

Breast tenderness

Cervical dysplasia

Cold hands and feet as a symptom of thyroid dysfunction

Copper excess

Decreased sex drive

Depression with anxiety or agitation

Dry eyes

Early onset of menstruation

Endometrial (uterine) cancer

Fat gain, especially around the abdomen, hips, and thighs

Fatigue

Fibrocystic breasts

Foggy thinking

Gallbladder disease

Hair loss

Headaches

Hypoglycemia

Increased blood clotting (increasing risk of strokes)

Infertility

Irregular menstrual periods
Irritability
Insomnia
Magnesium deficiency
Memory loss
Mood swings
Osteoporosis
PMS
Polycystic ovaries
Premenopausal bone loss
Prostate cancer
Sluggish metabolism
Thyroid dysfunction mimicking hypothyroidism
Uterine cancer
Uterine fibroids
Water retention, bloating
Zinc deficiency

❧ THE CAUSES OF ESTROGEN DOMINANCE

Strictly speaking, it's possible that we—men, women, and children—are all suffering a little from estrogen dominance, because there is so much of it in our environment. You would have to virtually live in a bubble to escape the excess estrogens we're exposed to through pesticides, plastics, industrial waste products, car exhaust, meat, soaps, and much of the carpeting, furniture, and paneling that we live with indoors every day. You may have on-and-off sinus problems, headaches, dry eyes,

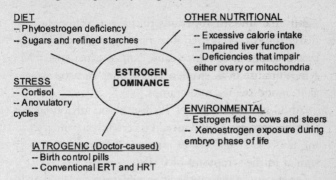

Figure 3.1. Potential Causes of Estrogen Dominance

asthma, or cold hands and feet, for example, and not know to attribute them to your exposure to xenohormones. Over time the exposure will cause more chronic problems, such as arthritis and premenopause symptoms, and may be a direct or indirect cause of cancer.

Figure 3.1 depicts the various sources and causes of estrogen dominance.

What makes estrogen dominance most noticeable in a premenopausal woman is a lack of ovulation. As early as her mid-twenties a woman may not ovulate during some of her monthly menstrual cycles. Ovulation refers to the time when an ovarian follicle releases an ovum (egg) that travels down the fallopian tube toward the uterus. After releasing the ovum, the emptied follicle becomes the corpus luteum that makes progesterone. This is the primary way that a premenopausal woman makes progesterone. If you don't ovulate, you won't make progesterone in any significant amount. You can still have a seemingly normal menstrual cycle even if you haven't ovulated, but the lack of progesterone may cause you to experience PMS symptoms such as swollen and tender breasts, weight gain, mood swings, and cramps.

Although the causes of PMS can't be attributed entirely to estrogen dominance, it is certainly a primary factor, and the symptoms of estrogen dominance are very similar to the symptoms of PMS.

There are many causes of anovulatory cycles, that is, menstrual cycles when a woman doesn't ovulate. One common cause is stress. The wisdom of the human body evolving over time dictates that a female body under stress may not be the best environment for a pregnancy. The types of stress most likely to induce anovulatory cycles are heavy exercise and extremely low calorie intake such as dieting, but any type of stress will do it, including emotional stress. Dr. Hanley has found that women who combine careers with raising a family and women who have extremely competitive and demanding corporate jobs also tend to have more anovulatory cycles. She has also seen women stop ovulating when they are in a physically or emotionally abusive relationship and when they have been through a serious illness.

The combination of estrogen dominance and stress can create a self-perpetuating cycle where stress causes estrogen dominance, which then causes insomnia and anxiety, which pulls on the adrenal glands, which then creates more estrogen dominance. A woman who has been caught in this type of cycle for a few years will find herself in a constant state of "wired but tired" (or "tired but wired"), which will eventually result in dysfunctional adrenal glands, blood sugar imbalances, and debilitating fatigue that may be diagnosed as chronic fatigue syndrome. One of our goals in this book is to help you identify a cycle like this and unwind it before it goes so far that you are debilitated.

Xenohormone exposure during embryo life damages ovarian follicles and leads to follicle failure later in life. This is probably a primary cause of anovulatory cycles in premenopausal women and a cause of the epidemic of infertility we're seeing in women of that age. The combined effects of low progesterone caused by anovulatory cycles and exposure to estrogenic xenohormones are more than enough to put the average woman into a state of estrogen dominance. Over time this will create a cycle of premenopause syndrome that may include PMS, fibrocystic breasts, fibroids, irregular periods, or endometriosis.

Another common cause of estrogen dominance and much misery is hysterectomy, or removal of the uterus, which creates surgically induced menopause. Even when the ovaries are left intact, their blood supply is severely compromised by hysterectomy, and they usually stop functioning altogether within two years of the removal of the uterus. But women who have a hysterectomy get a double whammy from conventional medicine, thanks to the common and extremely misguided practice of prescribing only estrogen and no progesterone to women with hysterectomies. Between estrogen-only hormone replacement therapy, estrogen made in fat cells, and environmental estrogens, estrogen dominance is almost guaranteed.

Supplemental estrogen in a woman who doesn't need it, or who has no progesterone to balance it, leads to more water retention, breast swelling, fibrocysts in the breasts, headaches, depression, fat storage, gallbladder problems, and hormone-related cancers; in women who still have their uteruses, heavier periods can result.

✦ THE TRUTH ABOUT ESTROGEN RESEARCH

The closer you get to menopausal age, the harder conventional medical doctors will try to push estrogen on you. We hope you'll resist these biased efforts and make an educated decision about whether or not to use estrogen.

If you believe everything you hear or read in the media, you would think that estrogen is a panacea for nearly everything, including all of the symptoms of aging, and especially Alzheimer's disease, osteoporosis, and heart disease. Clever marketing and advertising strategies on the part of the multibillion-dollar drug companies have created a surreal state of affairs around estrogen research. Dozens of small, unpublished studies done in obscure places by unknown scientists on the merits of estrogen appear with much regularity and fanfare in the popular media. These are likely to be one of the thirty- to sixty-second sound bites of so-called medical news that you frequently see on your local TV news and read in your local newspaper. These reports are generated by drug companies. The information is unquestioned and unexamined by the media that regurgitates them back to you. To them, it is simply "health news" filler that keeps major advertisers happy (especially the drug company executives, who spend billions of dollars every year). Superficial, unresearched articles indirectly promoting drug company products also appear in dozens of mainstream magazines that are supported by drug company dollars. We can't encourage you strongly enough to be extremely skeptical and wary of the medical information you get from mainstream media.

One of the most bizarre consequences of medical information created by drug companies is the use of the word *estrogen* to mean hormone replacement therapy. The miracles of estrogen are touted in the information released to the media, but if you go back and read the study the research was based on, you will almost always find that the women were also taking synthetic progesterone-like compounds called progestins. This is deliberately misleading and is an attempt to underplay the dangers of estrogen. In other words, if you keep reading about all the wonderful results gained from using estrogen, eventually you'll be convinced that it is indeed a miracle drug. But in truth, most of the results you read about also involved the use of a progestin or a progesterone or may have been due to the fact that women who are prescribed estrogen tend to have a healthier lifestyle to begin with than those who aren't.

Let's take the studies on Alzheimer's disease and estrogen as an example. It is already well known that women of higher socioeconomic status and with more education have a lower rate of Alzheimer's disease, but this has not been factored in to any of the studies done to date, nor have there been any long-term, double-blind studies. Moreover, there has been no reliable accounting of which women were also taking a progestin with their estrogen and which women had an intact uterus—all confounding factors.

There's no doubt that estrogen has an excitatory effect on the brain and that it can improve memory, which would improve the symptoms of Alzheimer's disease. But long-term estrogen dominance can have the opposite effect on the brain, creating chronic overexcitation, which leads to cell death, an increased risk of blood clots (and therefore strokes), and imbalances in cellular fluids, which can cause headaches.

Estrogen is a wonderful and useful hormone to be used with great care only when necessary, in very small amounts, in its natural form (meaning that it is identical to the estrogens made by your body). The primary symptoms of true estrogen deficiency are hot flashes, night sweats, and vaginal dryness. An estrogen deficiency can also cause fatigue, memory problems, and foggy thinking, but estrogen dominance can cause the same symptoms. The bladder contains estrogen receptors and is sensitive to estrogen. An estrogen deficiency can cause or worsen bladder and urinary tract problems. Many of the hormonal contraceptives are known for causing chronic urinary tract problems, possibly because they block the action of your own estrogen.

Estrogen deficiency symptoms can often be relieved with lifestyle changes such as an increase in exercise and dietary changes; by using some natural progesterone, which is a precursor to estrogen; or with some herbs that have estrogenic properties. All of these solutions will be covered in more detail later in the book.

Excess estrogen is processed through the liver, so if your liver function is compromised by drinking too much alcohol or using prescription drugs, for example, your estrogen levels will be higher. This is why estrogen dominance symptoms can sometimes be cleared up simply by making some healthy lifestyle changes.

If you do need to supplement some estrogen, you can use a natural estrogen in a cream, a patch, or a pill. Estrogen, and especially estriol, is not as easily absorbed through the skin as progesterone is, so it tends to work equally well orally or transdermally. If you have whole-body symptoms such as hot flashes and night sweats, you can use estrogen daily and experiment to find the smallest dose that will maintain balance. If you're just experiencing vaginal dryness, very small amounts of estrogen cream used vaginally once or twice a week should effectively stop it. Estriol, which may also help protect against breast cancer, is especially effective in maintaining healthy vaginal mucosa and protecting against urinary tract infections when used as a vaginal cream.

There is absolutely no doubt that estrogen can be very helpful to women who are truly estrogen deficient and that using an estrogen patch or cream for a few years around the age of menopause may help slow bone loss. In fact, a number of studies have found that heavier women who are producing more estrogen in their fat cells have better bone density.

But taken in even the slightest excess, estrogen becomes a potent promoter of cancer, and you need to always have that in the back of your mind when you're using it. This also makes it extremely important that you always use estrogen with progesterone to create hormonal balance. The tendency of conventional medical doctors to blithely prescribe estrogen for any type of premenopausal or menopausal symptom is irresponsible, dangerous, and has tragic consequences.

In the next chapter you'll find out how progesterone neutralizes the dangers of estrogen, how widespread its beneficial effects are in the body, and why you want to keep your distance from the synthetic progestins, even in birth control pills.

Chapter 4

--- ❖ ---

Progesterone and Progestins: The Great Protector and the Great Impostors

"It's as if my body breathed a big sigh of relief."

"My life is back on track and my symptoms are gone."

"I thought my ability to think clearly was gone for good, but it's back and better than ever."

"I had a second ultrasound and the fibroid is half the size it was six months ago. My doctor says I don't need to have a hysterectomy after all."

"My PMS and tender breasts are a thing of the past. And I'm in control of my emotions the week before my period."

"After three months on progesterone, folic acid, and vitamin B6 I am no longer testing positive for cervical dysplasia."

"Since I began using progesterone cream I haven't had one migraine headache."

"I've lost eleven pounds and I think most of it was water weight. I no longer feel like a balloon."

"I can sleep again and I'm much less moody and anxious."

"We just wanted to let you know that we had a healthy baby boy."

These are the kinds of letters, faxes, and phone calls that Dr. Lee and Dr. Hanley receive every day from women whose premenopausal symptoms cleared up after they began using a natural progesterone cream. It may sound too good to be true, but it's merely a case of supplying the body with what it needs to maintain balance. You've read about how out of balance our estrogenic environment has become; it's no wonder women are feeling much better when they use some progesterone.

Here is a letter typical of those that Dr. Lee receives every day:

My name is Erica. I will be 43 in August. When I turned 40, three months later I had my first hot flash. The hot flashes got worse and more frequent. I started monitoring my periods for about a year.

My periods had always been very regular. During that year my periods would be five days early, four days late, and so on. Then the night sweats started; the short-term memory loss and the insomnia were horrible. Also my blood pressure would be high certain times of the month. I've always had good blood pressure. About four months before I found your book, I had lost interest in sex.

The day I finally found a doctor who told me I was definitely perimenopausal, I had been on my period for 13 days. He put me on a low-dose birth control pill to help me with my symptoms. It did help me with my symptoms but also gave me horrible side effects. I gained weight, my breasts were so sore I could not go without a bra. . . . I had gas pains in my lower abdomen all the time. I had huge blood clots with my periods, and I was bloated all of the time. I took the pill for about a year, then it wasn't working for me anymore. The hot flashes came back, the night sweats came back, and the insomnia was unbearable. My doctor gave me a stronger birth control pill. I took them for two cycles and could not stand it any longer. My side effects were worse than before.

At this point I found your book. I read it, and I highlighted a lot that pertained to me and kept going back to it. I could not put your book down. I went right to the health food store and bought the progesterone cream. I stopped taking the pill and started the cream on Christmas morning, which turned out to be the 12th day of my cycle. That was the best Christmas present I ever had.

The first thing I noticed when I started using the cream was that my libido was back almost immediately. I don't have night sweats anymore, I don't get the short-term memory loss, I have been able to lose weight. The most amazing thing is, I no longer have any PMS symptoms before my period. I don't even know that it's coming anymore. My breasts do not hurt at all, not even before my period.

My mom also has your book. I loaned my book to my sister who has had a hysterectomy, and she has just gone out and bought her first tube of progesterone cream. I tell everyone about it, co-workers and friends. Finding your book Dr. Lee was the best thing that could have ever happened to me. Thank you!

Unlike estrogen, progesterone is not a generic name but rather is the name of the hormone produced by the corpus luteum after ovulation (see figure 4.1) and in smaller quantities by the adrenal gland. It is synthesized in humans in a biochemical pathway leading from cholesterol to pregnenolone to progesterone. In turn, progesterone is the precursor of corticosteroids and testosterone. Progesterone is also synthesized, in copious amounts, by the placenta during pregnancy.

Progesterone is a specific molecule made by mammals and has multiple roles in your body. It affects every tissue

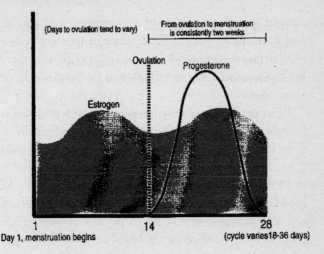

Figure 4.1. Days of Menstrual Cycle
Note that progesterone is measured in nanograms (ng) and estro-
gen is measured in picograms (pg) which is 1/1,000 of a
nanogram. In other words, estrogen is a much more potent hor-
mone than progesterone. If this diagram were to scale, the proges-
terone line would fill a page twice this size, and the estrogen line
would be nearly invisible at the bottom of the chart. Also notice
that ovulation may occur anytime from days 3 to 14 of your men-
strual cycle, but that the time between ovulation and menstrua-
tion is consistently two weeks.

in your body including the uterus, cervix, and vagina, the
endocrine (hormonal) system, brain cells, fat metabolism, thyroid hormone function, water balance, periph-
eral nerve myelin sheath synthesis, bone cells, energy
production and thermogenesis, the immune system,

survival and development of the embryo, and growth and development of the fetus. Though referred to as a sex hormone, progesterone conveys no specific secondary sex characteristics and as such cannot be called a male or female hormone.

Progesterone is a highly fat-soluble compound that is absorbed exceedingly well when applied transdermally or onto the skin. According to hormone researcher David Zava, Ph.D., progesterone is by far the most lipophilic, or fat loving, of the steroid hormones. It circulates in the blood, carried by fat-soluble substances such as red blood cell membranes. Some 70 to 80 percent of ovary-made progesterone is carried on red blood cells and thus is not measured by serum or plasma blood tests. This progesterone is available to the body for use and readily filters through the saliva glands into saliva where it can be measured accurately. The remaining 20 to 30 percent of progesterone in the body is protein bound and is found in the watery blood plasma where it can be measured by serum or plasma blood tests. However, only 1 to 9 percent of this progesterone is available to the body for use. That is why saliva testing is a far more accurate and relevant test than blood tests in measuring bioavailable progesterone.

The fall of progesterone levels at menopause is proportionately much greater than the fall of estrogen levels. Although estrogen falls only 40 to 60 percent from baseline on average, progesterone can decline to nearly zero. Furthermore, anovulatory cycles will cause low progesterone levels on and off throughout the premenopausal years.

One of progesterone's most important and powerful roles in the body is to balance or oppose estrogen. When our progesterone levels are in balance, excess estrogen is better handled. Some effects of excess estrogen as compared with the opposing effects when progesterone levels are adequate follow.

Estrogen Effects	Progesterone Effects
Creates proliferative endometrium	Maintains secretory endometrium
Causes breast stimulation	Protects against fibrocystic breasts
Increases body fat	Helps use fat for energy
Increases salt and fluid retention	Acts as natural diuretic
Causes depression and headaches	Acts as natural antidepressant
Interferes with thyroid hormone	Facilitates thyroid hormone action
Increases blood clotting	Normalizes blood clotting
Decreases sex drive	Restores sex drive
Impairs blood sugar control	Normalizes blood sugar levels
Causes loss of zinc and retention of copper	Normalizes zinc and copper levels
Reduces oxygen levels in all cells	Restores proper cell oxygen levels

Estrogen Effects	Progesterone Effects
Increases risk of endometrial cancer	Prevents endometrial cancer
Increases risk of breast cancer	Helps prevent breast cancer
Slightly restrains osteoclast function	Stimulates osteoblast bone building
Reduces vascular tone	Restores normal vascular tone
Increases risk of endometrial disorders	Functions as precursor of corticosteroids
Creates progesterone receptors	Increases sensitivity of estrogen receptors
Increases risk of prostate cancer	Helps prevent prostate cancer
	Allows embryo to survive

✢ PROGESTERONE ROLES AND RECEPTORS

Progesterone is a central factor in the biosynthesis of other hormones, but it also has many other important functions in the body, as shown in figure 4.2.

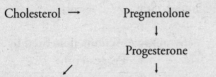

Cholesterol → Pregnenolone
↓
Progesterone
↓

Biosynthetic pathways	Reproductive Effects	Intrinsic Effects
Androstenedione	Maintains secretory endometrium	Acts as mild diuretic
Testosterone		Helps use fat for energy
Estrone, estradiol, estriol	Aids in survival of embryo	Acts as natural antidepressant
All cortisol and corticosteroids	Aids in development of fetus throughout gestation	Helps thyroid hormone action
Aldosterone		Normalizes blood clotting
	Increases libido	Helps normalize blood sugar levels
		Normalizes zinc and copper levels
		Maintains proper cell oxygen levels
		Protects against breast cysts
		Protects against breast cancer
		Protects against endometrial cancer
		Moisturizes skin (topically)
		Counteracts estrogen side effects

Figure 4.2. The Multiple Roles of Natural Progesterone
Progesterone has important effects throughout the body, and on all systems of the body, including acting as a precursor to the steroid hormones, maintaining pregnancy and other reproductive functions, and many intrinsic, or built-in, regulatory functions.

Hormones convey their messages only where and when receptors for them are available. The multiple roles of progesterone are illustrated by the range of progesterone receptors throughout the body. Based on our current knowledge, here are the areas of the body where progesterone receptors are found.

Sites	Symptoms/Actions Benefited by Progesterone
Brain	
Limbic brain	Emotion/psychological symptoms, epilepsy
Hypothalamus	Menstrual cycle (gonadotrophin-releasing hormone), hot flashes, and libido (ventral medial nucleus)
Preoptic area	Libido (sex drive)
Ventral tegmental area	Libido (sex drive)
Meninges	Headaches
Pituitary	Gonadotropic hormones
Peripheral nerves (Schwann's cells)	Myelin repair
Respiratory system	
Nasopharyngeal mucosa	Rhinitis, sore throat, sinusitis, pharyngitis, laryngitis
Lungs	Asthma
Skin	Dryness and thinning, various dermatoses, alopecia
Eyes	Glaucoma

Sites	Symptoms/Actions Benefited by Progesterone
Breast	Breast lesions, cell maturation, and replication rate
Fallopian tubes	Congestion, dysfunction
Uterus (fundus)	Endometrial diseases, myomata
Uterus (cervix)	Cervical mucous changes
Testes	Testosterone production
Adrenal glands	Corticosteroid production

❖ THE MULTIPLE ROLES OF ❖ PROGESTERONE IN A NUTSHELL

Procreation

- Maintains the secretory endometrium (the lining of the uterus) for nurturing a possible fertilized ovum
- Makes the cervical mucus accessible by sperm
- Allows embryo to survive
- Stops ovulation by the other ovary
- Prevents immune rejection of the developing baby, which carries the "foreign" DNA of the father
- Allows for full development of the fetus throughout pregnancy
- Facilitates the use of body fat for energy during pregnancy

- Activates osteoblasts to increase new bone formation
- Allows development of baby without secondary sexual development
- Increases libido at time of ovulation

Hormone Precursor Effects

- Functions as primary precursor for all adrenal corticosteroids
- Functions as primary precursor for estrogens
- Functions as primary precursor for testosterone produced by testes in males

Intrinsic Effects

- Protects against breast fibrocysts
- Protects against endometrial, breast, ovarian, and prostate cancer
- Normalizes blood clotting (excess estrogen causes abnormal blood clotting) and protects against strokes
- Acts as a natural diuretic (excess estrogen causes water retention)
- Acts as a natural antidepressant and relieves anxiety
- Helps normalize blood sugar levels
- Restores proper cell oxygen levels (estrogen depletes cell oxygen levels)
- Normalizes zinc and copper levels

- Helps thyroid hormone function (estrogen interferes with thyroid hormone use)
- Helps use fat for energy (estrogen converts food energy into fat)
- Stimulates osteoblast-mediated new bone formation (reverses osteoporosis)
- Maintains normal cell membrane functions
- Restores normal sensitivity of estrogen receptor
- Has beneficial anti-inflammatory effects
- Is useful in some cases of seizure disorder (epilepsy)
- Reduces incidence of autoimmune disorders
- Is thermogenic (raises body temperature)
- Helps metabolize body fat for energy production
- Helps prevent hypertension
- Prevents yeast (candida) infections at physiologic doses
- Increases immunoglobin E (Ig-E) to help prevent sinus, respiratory, and vaginal infections and allergic reactions

Clearly progesterone is a hormone that you want a good supply of—in the right balance, of course. We'll give you detailed instructions on how to decide if you need progesterone, and how to use it, in chapter 16.

✤ THERE CAN BE TOO MUCH OF A GOOD THING

Although it would be difficult to create a onetime overdose of progesterone, it is possible to use too much progesterone over time. What happens when too much progesterone is used? The pattern is similar to creating other types of hormone balance: The benefits conveyed in normal, physiologic doses when there is a deficiency are reversed when too much is used. (A physiologic dose mimics what the body would make if it was healthy and balanced, as opposed to a pharmacologic dose—or megadose—which is how most drugs are used.) Excess progesterone exhausts or otherwise reduces receptor sensitivity so that its benefits are often lost.

At physiologic doses, progesterone enhances some normal immune defenses in the body while at the same time it stops nonself-tissue rejection within the uterus, necessary for the survival of the embryo should there be one. (Organ transplant specialists are studying this attribute of progesterone.) But at excessively high doses, these benefits of progesterone may be lost or reversed.

In the breast, progesterone plays an important role during pregnancy in developing the specialized tissue that allows lactation. Women who use too much progesterone may find their breasts are considerably enlarged by this effect. Although this may sound like a positive attribute to some women, using excessive progesterone to create large breasts is not recommended, as the effect will wear off when progesterone levels return to normal, possibly resulting in sagging breasts (an effect familiar to women who have nursed their babies).

Brain cells concentrate progesterone to levels twenty times higher than serum levels. In the brain, progesterone reduces brain cell excitability. At normal levels, this allows people to focus, or concentrate, better. Moderately high levels can be used effectively as an anticonvulsant. In the 1950s, it was recommended for epilepsy. A recent study done in Sweden showed that women with catamenial epilepsy (epilepsy that is more severe premenstrually) have consistently low progesterone and high estrogen levels. Animal studies of epilepsy have consistently shown that progesterone is directly anticonvulsive and that some of its metabolites have a stabilizing effect on the nervous system. The fact that catamenial epilepsy doesn't improve during pregnancy when progesterone levels are high suggests that high estrogen levels also play an important role in seizures.

If progesterone levels are higher than normal for more than six months, people become mentally lethargic and even depressed. This happens most often with oral, micronized progesterone and high-dose creams. Fortunately, the effects of using too high a dose of progesterone over time is reversible by returning to normal levels of progesterone.

Progesterone has been used in studies to prevent endometrial hyperplasia (excessive growth of the uterine lining), to stop menstruation, and to stop ovulation (a rise in progesterone is what signals the other ovary not to ovulate), and it has been approved by the FDA for treating amenorrhea (lack of menstruation). However, when progesterone is taken orally, it is absorbed and transported to the liver where 80 to 90 percent of it is converted to metabolites that are meant to be excreted from the body. Only 10 to 20 percent of the oral dosed progesterone gets to the body as progesterone. That is why doctors using oral progesterone have to prescribe doses as high as 200 mg per day to get results. Since some of these metabolites do enter general circulation and have undesirable side effects, oral dosing should be avoided.

Transdermal (via skin) creams are the safest and most effective way to get the proper physiologic dose of progesterone.

Dr. David Zava reports that women who use too much progesterone experience significant abdominal bloating and discomfort, which he believes is due to a suppressive effect on the digestive system. He has also seen evidence that excessive progesterone may drive cortisol levels too high, resulting in cortisol-excess symptoms such as increased appetite and weight gain, particularly around the abdomen.

For detailed information on how to gauge your progesterone dosage, please see chapter 16.

✦ PROGESTINS

After seeing three doctors who couldn't help her, Stephanie flew from the Midwest to see Dr. Hanley. Nearly a year before, her gynecologist had talked her into using a birth control method that involved implanting capsules containing a progestin in her upper arm. The idea was that the progestin was slowly released into the bloodstream over a period of many months, providing a convenient and reliable method of contraception.

For a few months everything had seemed fine. Then Stephanie began to spot unpredictably, and pretty soon she was spotting or bleeding a little bit nearly all of the time. She called her doctor, who told her that the bleeding was normal and not to worry about it, but she worried anyway, and found it was interfering with her sex life. Stephanie also began having difficulty sleeping, and within six months was unable to sleep for more than four or five hours a night, though she always felt tired and wished she could sleep more. She was occasionally having severe abdominal pain that she said felt like a combination of a terrible muscle cramp and a branding iron inside. When she called her doctor's office and asked for an appointment to have the implants taken out, the doctor got on the phone and told her that her insomnia was not caused by the progestin, and he talked her into leaving them in. Finally, after nine difficult months, Stephanie demanded that the implants be removed. The removal, which was supposed to be painless and not leave any scars, left her arm swollen and sore for days with a scarred and lumpy area the size of a half-dollar. Worst of all, her symptoms still didn't go away. She still couldn't sleep and was still bleeding.

Dr. Hanley put Stephanie on a cleansing and detoxification program that supported her liver, and sent her to a plastic surgeon to find out if all of the progestin capsules had been removed. He found two of them had been left in her arm. Once those were out the constant bleeding stopped, but her menstrual cycles still weren't normal, and she was still having trouble sleeping. After giving Stephanie a couple of months to clear the progestins out of her system, Dr. Hanley put her on some natural progesterone cream and gave her some herbs to help her sleep. They also worked out a diet and exercise program designed to detoxify her body and bring back her sleep rhythms. Within three months Stephanie was back to normal—and using a diaphragm for birth control.

Progestins are synthetic chemical analogs of progesterone, meaning they have some progesterone-like effects. They are chemical alterations of the progesterone molecule and are not the same as progesterone (see figure 4.3). Since the 1950s, progestins have become widely used in birth control pills and in hormone replacement therapy (HRT).

Progesterone is not marketed by the big drug companies for hormone replacement therapy because it is a natural substance. They can't patent it, can't have exclusive use of it, and can't charge you outrageous prices for it. (Recently some drug companies have come out with natural progesterone in patentable delivery systems—an oral micronized progesterone and a vaginal gel.) It's theoretically possible that progesterone cream could be used for birth control, but appropriate studies of dose and efficacy have not been done.

Progestins are commonly made from progesterone or testosterone, which results in varying effects, including

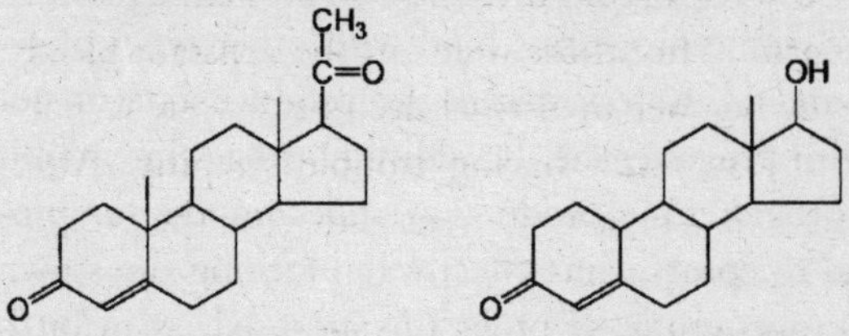

Progesterone
(pregn-4-ene-3,20-dione)

19-Nortestosterone
(17beta-hydroxy-19-norandrost-4-en-3-one)

Figure 4.3. Molecular Structure of Progesterone and 19-Nortestosterone

These molecular diagrams of progesterone and 19-nortestosterone, a common progestin (synthesized from testosterone) used in birth control pills, illustrate their differences. It should be obvious that 19-nortestosterone is not progesterone. Yet many medical writers refer to such progestins as progesterone or types of progesterone. Such references are semantic errors and lead to great confusion in the minds of physicians who read them.

an array of potential side effects that range from unpleasant to harmful. The most common side effects of taking progestins are bloating (particularly in the abdomen), painful breasts, mood swings, fatigue, depression, rashes and dry skin, dry itchy eyes, weight gain, diarrhea, constipation, anxiety, and joint and muscle pain.

Progestins are not found anywhere in nature and are foreign to human bodies. In general, they are more potent than progesterone. In addition to their potential for undesirable side effects, they fail to provide the full spectrum of natural progesterone's benefits. Unlike real progesterone, some progestins bind with other types of receptors and with testosterone to produce effects not found with progesterone. In addition, progestins inhibit normal progesterone production and compete for progesterone receptors, thus effectively blocking one's own natural progesterone. If progestins are used, as in birth control pills, supplementing with natural progesterone will have little or no benefit.

❧ AVOID HEART ATTACKS BY AVOIDING PROGESTINS

It is well known that premenopausal women rarely get heart attacks, but after menopause women quickly catch up to the rate common to men. Even after menopause a woman's heart attack profile is different from a man's because women suffer from fewer heart attacks caused by clogged arteries and more caused by spasms of the heart muscles.

In a landmark study by K. Miyagawa and associates, researchers at the Oregon Regional Primate Research Center set out to study the effect of hormones on coronary spasms. They removed the ovaries from 18 rhesus monkeys (used because their hearts most closely approximate human hearts) to simulate menopause and then put them on estrogen. Then 6 of the monkeys were put on natural progesterone, and 6 were put on medroxyprogesterone (Provera). Four weeks later the monkeys were injected with chemicals intended to cause coronary spasm. The monkeys that were on medroxyprogesterone and estrogen suffered an unrelenting spasm that would have caused death had they not been injected within minutes with a drug that reversed the spasm. The monkeys that had been treated with natural progesterone quickly recovered normal blood flow.

These findings are echoed by work done at the Wake Forest University Bowman School of Medicine in Winston-Salem, North Carolina, by M. R. Adams. In their research with monkeys, heart disease, and hormones Adams and his colleagues have shown that medroxyprogesterone "can obliterate the beneficial effect of estrogen therapy on the progression of coronary artery atherosclerosis," which is clogging of the arteries.

At London's National Heart and Lung Institute, in a study led by Peter Collins, women on different combinations of HRT were put on a treadmill. Once again, those who were using natural progesterone with estrogen could exercise significantly longer than those who took medroxyprogesterone.

For those of you who have doctors who are still telling you, your older sisters, or your mothers that progestins and progesterone are the same thing, the following table illustrates a side-by-side comparison of their effects. We always like to ask, "If progesterone and progestins are the same, why is it that an ample supply of progesterone is essential for a healthy pregnancy, while even tiny amounts of progestins are contraindicated during pregnancy because they cause birth defects?"

COMPARISON OF THE EFFECTS
OF PROGESTERONE AND PROGESTINS

Conditions	Natural (Real) Progesterone	Progestin
Increases sodium and water in body cells		✓
Causes loss of mineral electrolytes from cells		✓
Causes intracellular edema		✓
Causes depression		✓
Increases birth defect risks		✓
Causes facial hirsutism, loss of scalp hair		✓
Causes thrombophlebitis, embolism risk		✓
Decreases glucose tolerance		✓
Causes allergic reactions		✓
Increases risk for cholestatic jaundice		✓
Causes acne, skin rashes		✓
Protects against endometrial cancer	✓	✓
Protects against ovarian cancer	✓	
Protects against breast cancer	✓	
Normalizes libido	✓	

Conditions	natural (real) progesterone	progestin
Causes less hirsutism, regrowth of scalp hair	✓	
Improves lipid profile	✓	
Improves in vitro fertilization	✓	
Improves new bone formation	✓	modestly
Increases risk of coronary vasospasm		✓
Decreases risk of coronary vasospasm	✓	
Facilitates thyroid hormone action	✓	
Usually effective in treating PMS	✓	
Prevents implantation of fertilized ovum		✓
Is essential for successful pregnancy	✓	
Is essential for myelinization of nerves	✓	
Restores normal sleep patterns	✓	
Is a precursor of other steroid hormones	✓	
Is essential also for males	✓	

Chapter 5

How We Got into Xenohormone
Hell—and How to Get Out

Darcy was a forty-two-year-old woman who went to Dr. Hanley one fall, complaining of a multitude of symptoms. Dr. Hanley could tell when Darcy walked into her office that she was probably estrogen dominant: Her face had a red, flushed look to it; she was carrying some fat on her stomach and hips; and she had almost no hair on her arms. She told Dr. Hanley that she had gained almost fifteen pounds over the summer and couldn't figure out why. She was also finding that she became short of breath and tired out very easily, which upset her because she loved to garden and had two large dogs she liked to walk on the beach. She said she had recently tried to give one of her dogs a flea bath and had to sit down in the middle of it because she was so dizzy and tired. She was also having strange outbreaks of hives and rashes on her neck, chest, and back.

Dr. Hanley asked Darcy what kind of flea control she was using for her dogs. It was a potent pesticide that acts as a nerve poison in both humans and insects, not to mention dogs. In the small amounts present in a flea bath, it doesn't usually cause enough symptoms to be noticeable right away in humans and dogs, but Darcy had used it half a dozen times over the summer and the effects had accumulated. Her dogs were also wearing flea collars that contained a similar type of insecticide, and she'd had her house exterminated for fleas in the middle of the summer. She had also had her yard sprayed. That alone would have been enough to cause all of Darcy's symptoms, but she was also using potent pesticides, herbicides, and fungicides on her garden and liberal amounts of ant spray in the house. Her roses alone were doused with half a dozen chemicals.

"But I thought if they weren't safe they couldn't be sold!" she told Dr. Hanley.

Darcy is not alone in her ignorance of the dangers of pesticides and her zeal to get rid of everything that creeps, crawls, and bites. Pesticides are, for all practical purposes, unregulated. Thousands of chemicals that were sold before laws were made to protect consumers from unsafe substances are still on the shelves and have never been tested. Hundreds of new products come out every year, and few are adequately tested.

One popular herbicide widely advertised as so safe that a baby is shown sitting on grass treated with it, has never undergone thorough, long-term testing. Its manufacturer has done everything but thumb its nose at the U.S. Environmental Protection Agency (EPA). Finally it was put through some superficial testing, long after it had been on the market, but the scientist in charge of the testing was a recent former employee of the company that manufactures it. So the truth is that we really don't know whether it is safe or not. How could this be allowed to happen? Millions of innocent, unsuspecting people are using this product, assuming it is safe, when in all likelihood we will be looking back at the damage it is doing the way we are now looking back at DDT. Clearly our government is not going to protect us, and it is up to each one of us individually to act to protect ourselves, our families, and our communities. To use any type of pesticide, herbicide, or fungicide is to play Russian roulette with your health. It's not worth it.

Darcy had virtually bathed herself in xenohormones and nerve poisons that summer and was suffering from the effects. Xenohormones are substances not found in nature that have hormonal effects. We come into contact with many of these substances on a daily basis. Dr. Lee has done extensive research on the connection between xenohormones and hormone disruption in humans and has found much useful and thought-provoking information.

Common Sources of Xenohormones

- Solvents and adhesives
- Petrochemically derived pesticides, herbicides, and fungicides

- Car exhaust
- Emulsifiers found in soaps and cosmetics
- Nearly all plastics
- Industrial waste such as polychlorinated biphenyls (PCBs) and dioxins
- Meat from livestock fed estrogenic drugs to fatten them up
- Synthetic estrogens and progestins found in the urine of millions of women who take birth control pills and hormone replacement therapy (HRT), which is flushed down the toilet and eventually works its way into the food chain.

✦ GET SOLVENTS OUT OF YOUR LIFE

A common source of potent xenohormones is the type of chemicals called solvents. All organic solvents are volatile liquids at room temperature and are lipophilic. They enter the body with extreme ease through the skin, and they accumulate in lipid-rich tissues such as the brain, myelin (nerve sheath), and adipose (fat). In combination they may be additive, synergistic, or potentiated, meaning that their effects on the body could be vastly more potent and toxic in combination than separately.

Industries in which exposure to solvents is well known include automotive manufacturing and repair, paint and varnish manufacturing, the electronics industry, industrial cleaning, metal-part degreasing, and dry cleaning. In addition to work environments, exposure via hobbies must be considered. The use of most glues and fiberglass both involve exposure to solvents.

One of the most insidious routes of solvent exposure and toxicity is through fingernail polish and fingernail polish remover. Young girls are especially susceptible to the toxic and xenohormonal effects of solvents, and yet they are the ones most likely to have a dozen different shades of fingernail polish in the bedroom.

Some of the immediate effects of exposure to solvents include central nervous system (CNS) depression, which resembles fatigue or depression; psychomotor or attention deficits, which resemble incoordination and inability to focus; brain swelling (headaches); CNS capillary damage; and oxygen deprivation in the brain with possible permanent brain damage resulting in lowered cognitive abilities. Long-term exposure to solvents can cause mood disturbances such as depression, irritability, fatigue, anxiety, inability to focus, incoordination, and short-term memory loss. Solvents can also damage a developing fetus and should be studiously avoided in any amount by pregnant women.

✤ SOME GENERAL CLASSES OF ORGANIC SOLVENTS

Product labels should always be checked for the following.

Alcohols (e.g., methanol)
Aldehydes (e.g., acetaldehyde)
Aliphatic hydrocarbons (e.g., n-hexane)

Aromatic hydrocarbons (e.g., benzene)
Cyclic hydrocarbons (e.g., cyclohexane)
Esters (e.g., ethyl acetate)
Ethers (e.g., ethyl ether)
Glycols (e.g., ethylene glycol)
Halogenated hydrocarbons (e.g., carbon tetrachloride, trichlorethylene)
Ketones (e.g., acetone, methylethylketone)
Nitrohydrocarbons (ethyl nitrate)

All xenohormones should be considered toxic; the majority of them have estrogenic effects on both male and female bodies. (See figure 5.1.) They are extremely potent and are active in almost unbelievably small doses, and the petrochemically derived xenohormones are non-biodegradable, so they will continue to accumulate in the environment for as long as they are being manufactured. Xenohormones are fat soluble, so they pass easily through the skin, and they are cumulative as well, meaning they accumulate in the body over time.

Present environmental toxicity testing is usually restricted to signs of toxicity in the animal directly exposed to the toxic threat or to the presence of birth defects in their offspring. As we know from our experience with di-ethylstilbestrol (DES) and long-term animal studies, xenohormone toxicity may not show up until the midlife of the generation born after the generation exposed. That means that the present manner of testing will miss those effects. Furthermore, the dosages of the xeno-hormone causing the problem are so small that routine testing is unable to show it. For example, a single dose of dioxin at 0.064 µg/kg given to a pregnant female rat can result in the inhibition of masculinization in the male rat offspring. In other cases, the dose of the xenohormone causing malformations or sexual disruption may be in nanogram ranges. These doses are below the usual available testing sensitivity.

Moreover, the large number of petrochemical xenohormones released into the environment combined with their known persistence and lipophilic nature (making them easily absorbed through the skin and easily accumulating in fatty tissue) makes it inevitable that multiple endocrine disrupters accumulate in target tissues over time. It is common to find PCBs, dioxins, DDT, and a number of other organochlorine pesticides together in human breast tissue. This, of course, raises concern about their additive and synergistic effects.

This may explain why not all animals equally exposed to a given xenohormone produce offspring with similar effects. The damage that becomes evident is subject to at least three factors: the environmental exposure, genetic predisposition, and the time of life of the exposure.

Xenohormones create hormonal mayhem in all living creatures and are particularly damaging to ovaries and testes during the embryo stage. Chronic exposure results eventually in functional loss of ovarian follicles (decreased progesterone production) and Sertoli's cells in testes (decreased sperm production), leading to fertility problems, cancer, and general hormonal imbalance. Most xenohormones have estrogenic effects, which have

HO—⟨ ⟩—C=C—⟨ ⟩—OH

Diethylstilbestrol (DES)

DDT

Polychlorbiphenyl (PCB) structure

Bisphenol A

Examples of xeno-estrogens

Estradiol

Endogenous estrogen

Figure 5.1. Comparison of Several Xenoestrogens with Estradiol

created an epidemic of estrogen excess worldwide. There are several ways that xenohormones with estrogenic effects exert their influence on the body.

• Some combine with estrogen receptor sites and activate estrogenic action.
• Some appear to induce formation of extra estrogen receptors.
• Others may inhibit the ability of the liver to excrete estrogen.
• A few may occupy estrogen receptors and inhibit their action.

Animals serve as our early warning system about the toxic nature of our estrogenicized world. They are our canaries in the coal mine, and we need to pay attention to what is happening to them. The following list of physiologic and behavioral effects observed in wildlife exposed to xenohormones with estrogenic properties is alarming.

• Bill deformity and thin-shelled eggs in birds
• Grossly feminized reproductive tracts, even in male birds
• Abnormal nesting behavior
• Chemical castration of male birds
• Failed hatching of alligator eggs
• Abnormally high estrogen/testosterone ratios in female alligators

- Abnormally small penises and low levels of testosterone in male alligators
- Decreased sexual behavior in male rats and increased sexual behavior in female rats
- Inhibits estrogen receptors and causes masculinization of brain cells and sex-mounting behavior in female rats
- Abnormal production of vitellogenin (egg yolk protein) in male turtles
- Gender changes in turtles, fish, and mollusks
- "Burned-out" follicles in ovaries

Over two decades ago, it became apparent that daughters born of women given the synthetic estrogen DES during pregnancy carried an increased risk of malformations and cancer of the urogenital tract (vagina, cervix, ovary) as they reached maturity. In the past decade, it has become apparent that DES is merely one example of a large group of petrochemical compounds that all have potent estrogenic and other toxic properties in a wide variety of animal forms such as crustaceans, amphibians, fish, mammals, and birds. Such compounds include pesticides of all sort, solvents, plastics, and adhesives, with names such as dioxin, DDT, bisphenol A, PCBs, dieldrin, chlordane, and many others. Again, figure 5.1 shows the similarity between an estrogen molecule and various xenohormones that act as estrogens. Given the general environmental exposure to these pollutants, it seems likely that humans will be similarly affected.

In addition to the harmful effects on wildlife, now

well described in the book *Our Stolen Future* by Dr. Theo Colborn, Dr. Lee's research of the present epidemic of estrogen dominance and progesterone deficiency among women in industrialized countries leads to the conclusion that xenohormones are an important but unrecognized factor in our current epidemic of hormone imbalance. The working hypothesis is that ovaries are damaged by xenohormone exposure during one's embryonic development. If such damage occurs to birds, cougars, alligators, frogs, and fish, why not humans? When female animals are exposed to xenohormones during their pregnancy, female offspring are found to have obvious loss and dysfunction of ovarian follicles, affecting their reproductive ability later in life. The embryonic stage of life is the time when these tissues are most sensitive to the toxicity of xenohormones.

Functioning ovarian follicles are the primary source of progesterone in women. When damaged by xenohormones during early embryonic development, progesterone production later in life eventually declines, leading to luteal phase failure (early miscarriage), sleep disturbance, loss of normal libido, and estrogen dominance with symptoms such as fibrocystic breasts, water retention, increased fat deposition at hips and thighs, and an increased risk of estrogen-related cancers such as breast, ovary, and endometrium.

It is likewise recognized that xenohormones have toxic effects not clearly estrogenic. Prenatal exposure can cause multiple endocrine disruptions, anatomic deformities, and even intellectual impairment. In 1996 a remarkable study by J. L. Jacobson published in the *New England Journal of Medicine*, reported the correlation of intellectual impairment with in utero exposure to polychlorinated biphenyls (PCBs) among 212 children born of mothers living in western Michigan. The recruited families' diets were surveyed regarding consumption of Lake Michigan fish (known to be contaminated with PCBs), and, at birth, PCB levels in umbilical cord blood, mother's blood, and breast milk was measured. At age 11, those children with the highest prenatal exposure to PCBs were three times as likely to have low IQ scores and twice as likely to be at least two years behind in reading comprehension.

But what about exposure to xenohormones after birth? Xenohormones are fat soluble and nonbiodegradable. Continued exposure after birth should lead to progressively higher xenohormone tissue concentrations. If they are such potent estrogens, why doesn't it result in identifiable estrogen effects? The fact is, it does. In 1993 Devra Lee Davis of the Office of the Assistant Secretary for Health and coauthors representing multiple research centers summarized the evidence that xenohormones play a role in the induction of breast cancer, listing 78 references. The implications regarding xenohormones and hormone-dependent cancers are daunting.

In the April 1997 issue of *Pediatrics*, a study by M. E. Herman-Giddens reported a significant change in the onset of secondary sexual characteristics and menses in young girls age 3 through 12. Some 17,077 children were examined and their pubertal maturation rated by

225 clinicians. It was found that mean ages of breast development and pubic hair growth were 8.8 years for African American and 10 years for Caucasian girls. The prevalence of either pubic hair or breast development at age 5 was 5.7 percent for African American and 1.9 percent for Caucasian girls. By age 11, menses is established in 28 percent of African American and 13.4 percent of Caucasian girls. Taken together, these figures show that puberty is starting two years earlier now than previous standards of just ten to twenty years ago.

It is interesting—and odd—that the conclusion in the abstract by Herman-Giddens and colleagues merely advises practitioners to recognize the new norms and revise their criteria for referral of girls with precocious puberty. Referring to the premature pubertal changes as a new "norm" rather than an abnormality seems to miss the point. Since it is extremely unlikely that the change found is independent of some external cause such as environmental xenohormones, it would be more appropriate that the study should call for deeper investigation into the cause of the early pubertal changes. Should we not be calling for a meaningful reduction in the use of petrochemical xenohormones that are now threatening not only our health but in addition the normal development of all humankind?

The disturbing effects observed in humans of overexposure to xenohormones with estrogenic effects are summarized in the following list.

- Undersized penises and/or undescended testes in boys born to women exposed to PCBs
- A 50 percent decrease in sperm count since 1938
- An increased incidence of testicular and prostate cancer
- A potentiating or stimulating effect in breast cancer
- A potentiating or stimulating effect in endometriosis
- Endometrial cancer
- Cervical cancer in women whose mothers were given diethylstilbestrol (DES), a potent synthetic estrogen, during pregnancy
- Premenstrual syndrome (PMS)
- Fibrocystic breasts
- Postmenopausal osteoporosis
- Change in sexual orientation
- Estrogen dominance syndrome

Xenohormones adversely affect the developing reproductive system of both female and male embryos and fetuses. In particular, the follicles (ova bearers) of the ovaries of female embryos are damaged such that progesterone production is lost in early adult life. Such women will continue to produce estrogen and have menstrual cycles, but they will be deficient in progesterone and experience estrogen dominance. Dr. Lee's progesterone research of the past fifteen years shows the parallels between xenohormone effects and the symptoms of progesterone deficiency. As the current younger generations mature, we will almost certainly find that millions of them are reproductively crippled because of their excessive exposure to xenohormones in the womb. The following list itemizes health problems that have emerged or increased dramatically in incidence among women in the fifty years since petrochemicals were introduced.

1. Breast and uterine cancer incidences are increasing and are occurring at earlier ages.
2. Luteal phase failure is now the leading cause of early miscarriage and infertility.
3. Breast fibrocysts are more common.
4. PMS is increasing.
5. Osteoporosis in women is now more prevalent and more severe, and its onset is fifteen years or more before menopause, that is, before estrogen levels decrease.
6. Fat and water retention and numerous other signs and symptoms of estrogen dominance secondary to progesterone deficiency are epidemic in women.
7. Prolactinemia and prolactinoma (high prolactin levels and prolactin-producing pituitary tumors) are also inceasing dramatically and may also be related to petrochemical endocrine disruption.
8. Autoimmune disorders such as Sjögren's and lupus erythematosis are increasing in incidence and are correlated with estrogen dominance.

Xenohormones are ubiquitous in our diet and environment, and they are already recognized as the likely cause of the threatened die-off of a number of animal species in areas exposed to these toxic compounds. The fate of future generations of humanity may hinge on our ability to substantially decrease environmental contamination by the petrochemical xenohormones.

Clearly we need to minimize our exposure to these disruptive and destructive substances, both for the sake of our own health as well as the health of future generations. If you like a good cause to fight for, getting these chemicals out of our environment is one of the most important causes you could choose. Until some sanity is restored to our environment, here are some techniques for decreasing our exposure to these toxic chemicals.

1. Most obvious, but also most difficult: Drastically decrease reliance on pesticides of all sorts, including house sprays such as ant or fly spray, flea spray, lawn sprays, and garden sprays.

2. Eliminate or decrease consumption of foods most likely to be contaminated with these chemicals, such as meats, milk, and coffee. If you do eat red meat, poultry, eggs, meat, and fish, it should be organic and free of hormones and antibiotics. A primarily plant-based diet of fresh, unprocessed organically grown vegetables, fruits, nuts, and grains of all sorts is a foundation for good health and longevity for us and for the environment. Remember, it's up to you to request organic foods at your supermarket and to support your local farmers' market. We'll cover diet recommendations in detail in chapter 14.

3. Avoid exposure to solvents, plastics, and products such as cosmetics and soaps made with petrochemical-

based emulsifiers and spreaders, especially when you might be pregnant. Avoid surfactants such as nonoxynol (spermicides). This also means don't store or heat your food in plastics; don't wear plastic clothing (polyester comes to mind); and don't use air fresheners, fabric softeners, and scented laundry soaps.

4. Choose wood or stone tile floors rather than carpets. The glues and solvents in the backing of carpets will emit toxic molecules for several years. For the same reason, if you have a choice, avoid particle board and fake wood paneling when building a house.

5. Avoid all synthetic sex hormones.

Part II

WHEN YOUR BODY TALKS, LISTEN

What's Causing Premenopause Syndrome
Symptoms and How to Treat Them

Chapter 6

❖

How (and Why) to Keep Your Uterus and Save Your Cervix

*Y*our uterus, also known as your womb, is a remarkable and powerful muscular organ, ranging from the size of a fist in a woman who hasn't given birth, to the size of a watermelon in a woman in her last trimester of pregnancy. Any woman who has experienced monthly cramps, labor and childbirth, a deep orgasm that involves the uterus, or even the twinge from having a tissue sample taken during a pap smear has no doubt as to the power and muscularity of her uterus. And the uterus, it seems, has equal power to make life a joy or a misery.

Every month, for decades, the uterus builds up a glandular bloody lining—the endometrium—in response to hormonal signals and releases it in menstruation if the signals for pregnancy don't come. If a pregnancy does occur, the uterus gradually enlarges and becomes a perfect incubator for nine months of gestation.

It is primarily estrogen that stimulates the uterine lining to grow each month. As we age, our cells become increasingly susceptible to damage that can ultimately become cancer. This is particularly true of the growth-intensive tissue of the uterus. Considering the long-term and relatively rapid turnover of cells in the uterus, the frequent presence of estrogen, and estrogen's primary role in initiating and promoting cancer, you would think that uterine cancer in women would be common. After all, a lifetime of monthly exposure to estrogen would seemingly steeply raise the odds for mutated and damaged cells giving rise to cancer. And yet it is a remarkable fact that until doctors started giving women unopposed estrogen as hormone replacement therapy in the 1960s, uterine cancer (also called endometrial cancer) was extremely rare. In a woman's uterus, nature has created a powerfully protective anticancer milieu that almost always remains intact unless we throw it out of balance. When a woman does get endometrial cancer, the most common time for it to begin is about five years before the onset of menopause, when estrogen is still plentiful, but anovulatory cycles may be causing a chronic progesterone deficiency and therefore setting up estrogen dominance.

Endometrial cancer is one of the types of cancer we know most clearly how to prevent: Avoid unopposed estrogen.

❖ UTERINE ENLARGEMENT AND FIBROIDS

The uterus is one of the first organs to manifest symptoms when a woman's hormones are out of balance. Two of the most common uterine symptoms of premenopause syndrome are an enlarged uterus and uterine fibroids. Women with PMS often experience painful periods (dysmenorrhea) which are most often caused when the endometrial lining of the uterus extends into the muscular wall of the uterus (adenomyosis). When shedding of the endometrium occurs (menstruation), the blood is released into the muscular lining, causing severe pain. Conventional medicine treats this pain with nonsteroidal anti-inflammatory drugs (NSAIDs), such as ibuprofen, but ignores the underlying metabolic hormonal imbalance that caused it. The problem can be simply resolved by restoring proper progesterone levels, which restores normal growth and shedding of the endometrium.

Estrogen dominance causes the uterus to grow, and without the monthly balancing effect of progesterone it doesn't have the proper signals to stop growing. In some women this results in an enlarged uterus that presses on other organs, such as the bladder, and often on the digestive system, and generally causes discomfort and heavy menstrual bleeding. In other women estrogen dominance results in fibroids, which are tough, fibrous, noncancerous lumps that grow in the uterus. Some fibroids can grow to the size of a grapefruit or cantaloupe, causing constant bleeding and such heavy

menstrual periods that the blood loss is akin to hem-
orrhaging.

Fibroids always shrink at menopause, but the most
common course of action a doctor takes when a patient
comes in with a fibroid is to remove the uterus. The explanation given is that a fibroid is too difficult to remove
without irreversibly damaging the uterus. But in most
cases this is no longer true. If you do end up needing to
have a fibroid surgically removed, find a doctor who can
do it without removing your uterus with it. If you have
many small fibroids, it may be more difficult to remove
them. On the other hand, their smaller size may make it
easier to treat them without surgery.

Dr. Hanley treated a woman named Donna who, for
financial and emotional reasons, was determined not to
have a hysterectomy even though she had a huge fibroid
that was causing serious bowel and bladder problems.
Even after ending up in the emergency room she had refused surgery and had sought out Dr. Hanley, determined to find another way.

Dr. Hanley first talked to Donna about what was
going on in her life and discovered that right around the
time that she started to notice symptoms from the fibroid, she had finally extricated herself emotionally and
financially from a physically and sexually abusive relationship.

Since she was already in counseling and had a good
emotional support system of friends and family, the first
thing Dr. Hanley had her do was change her diet. Donna
had been living on milk, cheese, cottage cheese, and ice

cream. Dr. Hanley put her on a high fiber, vegetable-based diet along with some herbs to help detoxify her body and support her liver. Since it was an emergency situation, Dr. Hanley also gave her a shot of a synthetic drug called Lupron, which suppressed her ovary's production of hormones for three months, lowering her whole hormonal milieu, and also asked her to use a very small amount of progesterone cream. Within a few weeks her bowel and bladder problems were gone and Donna reported that she could feel her uterus begin to soften, indicating that the fibroid was shrinking. Just over seven months later, Donna was feeling like herself again, and her fibroid had shrunk to a manageable size.

Donna's story is unusual because most women will see a doctor and end up having a hysterectomy long before a fibroid gets large enough to cause severe pain and bladder problems, and most women do not have Donna's extreme fear of surgery. But Donna is a good example of how a woman can bring her body back into balance when she's willing to accept the challenge of working with herself in a focused way and has the dedication to stick with it.

Some 60 percent of women who reach age sixty-five will have a hysterectomy. For a small percentage of them it will relieve chronic pelvic pain and increase sexual pleasure. But for most women a hysterectomy results in reduced sexual pleasure, and it often does not cure pelvic pain. A hysterectomy in a premenopausal woman will also result in abrupt menopause and atrophy of the ovaries. It will increase her risk of heart disease and osteoporosis and will greatly increase her chances of having bladder problems such as incontinence and chronic urinary tract infections.

❧ WHY YOUR UTERUS IS A NUISANCE TO YOUR DOCTOR AND THE DRUG COMPANIES

What doctors aren't telling women is that giving them estrogen before menopause will cause a fibroid to grow—and that giving them estrogen after menopause (when it would naturally shrink) will likely cause it to continue to grow. What most doctors don't know about fibroids is that avoiding estrogen and using some natural progesterone cream will almost always shrink a fibroid enough to minimize or eliminate symptoms long enough to get to menopause, when it will normally shrink significantly enough to cease being a problem.

It's ironic that our conventional medical culture has evolved in such a way that a woman who has an enlarged uterus or a fibroid is considered to have a disease, and that her uterus is considered to be a liability, all because it has become a virtual requirement that your doctor prescribe Premarin and Provera to you when you reach menopause. If your doctor didn't feel so powerfully obliged to prescribe those drugs, your uterus would naturally shrink. Because he or she feels obliged to prescribe those drugs, your uterus becomes dangerous. Thus do drug company profits dictate medical education and practice.

Having a uterus also means that your doctor can't just

prescribe estrogen alone; he or she also is required to prescribe Provera (synthetic progesterone) to offset the cancer-causing effects of estrogen. The first attempts at
hormone replacement therapy (HRT) in the 1960s used
only estrogen, and this human experiment cost the lives
of thousands of women who died of uterine (endometrial) cancer in the 1960s and 1970s before it dawned on
the medical profession that unopposed estrogen was the
cause. It took another decade of intense public relations
and marketing campaigns to convince women that it was
safe once again to take HRT because they would now be
protected from cancer by the addition of a synthetic progestin to the mix, most commonly Provera.

But as Gail Sheehy so aptly described in her pioneering book *The Silent Passage* (see Bibliography), there aren't
too many drugs in the world that will make women feel
worse than Provera. Many women outright refuse to continue taking Provera when they experience its side effects
(something akin to severe, permanent PMS) and will even
risk cancer and take unopposed estrogen to avoid it. This
gives your doctor yet another reason to suggest that removing your uterus will solve a lot of problems. The
promise is that once your cancer-prone uterus is gone,
you're safe, and you can take only estrogen without the
Provera. The promise is that estrogen will save you from
heart disease, osteoporosis and Alzheimer's disease, so the
trade-off of losing your uterus is well worth it. Or so the
conventional wisdom goes. Unfortunately, these promises
aren't true. If you remove your uterus and take estrogen,
your troubles have only begun.

What a convoluted, tricky house of cards has been built around the belief that conventional HRT will save you from the ills of old age. All these lines of reasoning, assumptions, and belief systems are built on decades of clever but inherently dishonest advertising and marketing for estrogen. Premarin, the top-selling drug in America, has made your uterus a liability. The truth is that your uterus is not a liability to you; it is a liability to drug company profits.

Let's also briefly delve into the economics of a hysterectomy. Removal of your uterus is a very costly major surgery, with a long recovery time. After surgery, you will be visiting your doctor every six months or at least once a year to renew your hormone replacement prescription. This scenario gives both your doctor and a drug company a lifetime repeat customer, which is the dream of everyone in business, from the small entrepreneur to the corporate CEO. In other words, removing a woman's uterus is very, very good for business.

Furthermore, the unopposed estrogen that your doctor believes it is safe to prescribe now that you don't have a uterus will eventually lead to a long, expensive (but profitable to your doctor) sequence of pathologic conditions such as fibrocystic breasts, weight gain, water retention, hypertension (elevated blood pressure), blood clots, gallbladder disease, and breast or other hormone-dependent cancers. You have, in effect, become a cash cow for your doctor. Each and every disease you get from unopposed estrogen brings financial reward to your doctor. Behavior rewarded is behavior repeated.

Now let's look at the other choices. Removing a fibroid from a uterus takes a level of surgical skill, patience, and expertise that most ob-gyns don't have. It also takes longer and costs more, so insurance companies would rather not pay for it. Until fairly recently, very few ob-gyns were qualified to do the surgery, nor would the insurance companies cover it. If the ob-gyns can't do it themselves, they have to pass on your business to another surgeon. Or they can remove your uterus, which is a fairly simple and straightforward procedure (for the surgeon, not for you).

If you just have surgery to remove a fibroid, and you leave your uterus intact, after the surgery your doctor may not see you again except every few years for a pap smear.

Now let's say your doctor recommends using some progesterone cream. Well, you can buy that yourself, over the counter, and it's fairly easy to learn how to use it. That may be the last time you ever see that doctor, except to return for the ultrasound a year later, which will show that your fibroid has gone from the size of an orange to the size of a walnut.

The economics of these choices are extremely different for you and for your doctor. We aren't suggesting that you shouldn't ever have your uterus removed, because in rare cases that is necessary. But we are strongly recommending that you take into account the hidden agendas that exist in this type of a situation before making a decision, and that you make your decision based on what's best for you.

❧ HEALING THE UTERUS/FIBROIDS ❧

What to Do

- Use natural progesterone cream.*
- Eat a plant-based, fiber-rich diet (at least 20–30 g fiber per day).
- Take a liver-supporting and detoxifying herbal formula that includes some or all of the following herbs: *Bupleurum*, milk thistle (*Silybum marianum*), barberry or goldenseal, burdock root, yellow dock, dandelion root.
- Take a uterus-healing herbal formula that includes some or all of the following herbs: myrrh, red raspberry, cayenne, *Bupleurum*, yarrow, *Vitex* and lady's mantle (*Alchemilla mollis*).
- Use a castor oil pack 2 to 4 times a week (many books on herbal healing have instructions on how to make and use a castor oil pack).

What to Avoid

- Unopposed estrogen
- Dairy products
- Feed-lot meats (eat only range-fed, organic meats free of drugs and pesticide residues)
- Coffee (heavily sprayed with DDT)

*See chapter 16 for details on using natural progesterone cream.

❧ FLOODING, CLOTTING, AND CRAMPING

"I'm going through a Super Tampax and a heavy pad every hour! I can't even go to the grocery store without wondering if I'll have to leave with my jacket tied around my waist!"

"I had to pull the car over because I was sweating and shaking so much, and my cramps were so painful."

"I'm passing huge blood clots, am I okay?"

All of these women are okay in the sense that these symptoms don't necessarily mean serious illness. But they are signs of hormonal imbalance and a measure of the body's inability to smoothly down-regulate hormonal messages.

As they approach menopause, women tend to expect their menstrual cycles to become shorter, maybe even to be sporadic, with lighter bleeding. That may be the way it happened in the days before xenohormones and refined, processed foods, and that is certainly the preferable way to experience turning down the hormonal thermostat. But these days heavy bleeding is common, even in women who are still a decade from actual menopause. Sometimes heavy bleeding can be caused by a uterine fibroid, but it's equally likely that it's part of fluctuating premenopausal hormones and anovulatory cycles that allow unopposed estrogen to overstimulate the endometrium.

A menstrual period with very heavy bleeding is sometimes called flooding; these periods are often accompanied by short bouts of unusually painful cramping that mean large clots of blood are being passed. Both the heavy bleeding and the large clots can be scary for a woman who doesn't know it's "normal." Although flooding, cramping, and clotting may be a fairly common part of the premenopause experience these days, if we look at women's experiences over the past century, it probably can't be considered normal in a broader context, any more than it can be considered normal that girls are reaching puberty at the age of ten. It's a symptom of overexposure to estrogen, and it's possibly a symptom of exposure to xenohormones in the womb.

This flooding, cramping, and clotting is happening to so many thousands of women (most notably the premenopausal baby boomers), that there are ads about it on TV for "super" this and "heavy" that "feminine protection." These uncomfortable symptoms are at least partially due to an estrogen-dominant uterus. Heavy bleeding can occur when the uterus is exposed to relatively high levels of estrogen that stimulate excessive growth of the uterine lining. It's also possible that it is a result of mixed signals coming from the brain, from the adrenal glands in the form of stress hormones, and from a variety of xenohormones in the environment. A nutrient-poor diet can also contribute to heavier bleeding.

Carolyn DeMarco, M.D., says that the women she

❧ HEALING FLOODING, CRAMPING, ❧ AND CLOTTING

What to Do

- Maintain hormone balance as much as possible through diet, exercise, supplements, and, when needed, natural hormones.
- For cramping, use an herbal formula for menstrual cramps that contains some or all of the following herbs: cramp bark (*Viburnum opulus*), motherwort (*Leonurus cardiaca*), bleeding heart (*Corydalis*), wild yam (*Dioscorea*), skullcap, chamomile, blackhaw (*Viburnum prunifolium*). If your cramping occurs at a predictable time in your cycle, start using these herbs 2 to 4 days prior to the cramping.
- Take bioflavonoids to strengthen capillaries, 1,000 mg daily.

---

sees who have heavy bleeding have too much to do and are often overwhelmed with their lives. She also recommends checking iron levels with a blood test if heavy bleeding persists for more than a few months, and supplementing with a high-quality iron supplement if necessary.

If you have had pelvic pain or symptoms such as heavy bleeding prior to premenopause, please don't let your doctor rush or scare you into having a hysterectomy based only on these symptoms. Granted, they are a nuisance, but they will pass and they certainly aren't worth giving up an important organ without deeper consideration. If you're willing to do the work of making lifestyle changes and delving into the emotional side of your hormone imbalance, surgery can almost always be avoided.

❖ GETTING ACQUAINTED WITH YOUR CERVIX

In a very funny episode of a popular TV sitcom a menopausal woman is depressed about aging and in an attempt to reconnect her with her "inner crone," her daughter-in-law tries to get her to look at her cervix with a mirror. It wasn't so very long ago that not only did you not touch or look "down there," you didn't even talk about it. When you went for a pelvic exam, the doctor put your feet in the stirrups, pushed your knees up to your chin, and hid behind the blue sheet while he plunged a cold steel speculum up your vagina and "pinched" your cervix for a pap smear. As he pulled out the speculum and whipped off his rubber gloves he would point out the tissue box and leave the room, returning to talk only when you were fully wiped and dressed.

In most doctor's offices these days it's a little different. When you lie down on your back you might see a pleasant picture or piece of macramé on the ceiling. Any gynecologist or physician's assistant worth her salt will get you in the padded stirrups, put in the warmed speculum, and produce a mirror so that you can look at your own cervix. When she palpates your ovaries she'll explain what she's doing, and she might even tell you about how your particular uterus is large, or small, or tipped one way or another. So in some respects, we've come a long way.

Your cervix is technically a part of your uterus. It is the base of the uterus, the part that extends down into the vagina and through which a baby leaves the womb and begins to enter the world. It is one of the miracles of a woman's body that the opening of the cervix is so narrow that a finger can't penetrate it, until labor begins, when it dilates enough to allow the passage of a newborn infant.

If you put your finger into your vagina and feel the cervix, it feels similar to a nose or a chin. Just as the nose and chin come in many sizes and shapes, so does the cervix. Your cervix changes color, shape, and position depending on where you are in your menstrual cycle and your level of sexual arousal.

Women routinely visit a physician if for no other reason than to have a pap smear every few years. A pap smear is a test for cancerous or precancerous cells of the cervix that involves scraping some tissue from the opening of the cervix, putting it on a slide, and sending it to a laboratory. The pap smear will come back rated as a Class I through Class V. Class I is normal (benign), Class II is usually an irritation or inflammation, Class III is a true cervical dysplasia that can range from mild to serious, Class IV may be one of a variety of precancers or cancers, and Class V is a seriously invasive cancer. The problem with pap smears is that they have a very high rate (as much as 70 percent) of false positives, giving a more serious class rating than really exists, and a very high rate of false negatives, giving a less serious rating when there really is trouble. There is a new type of test available called the ThinPrep system that gives a significantly more accurate reading, but you're still subject to a lot of uncertainty if the test comes back "positive."

❖ DEMYSTIFYING CERVICAL DYSPLASIA

By far the most common "positive" or abnormal type of pap smear for which a doctor is likely to recommend surgery is known as cervical dysplasia, meaning abnormal cell growth in the cervix. When the doctor tells you this is a "precancerous" condition, it can be very scary, but you should know that you are almost always a long, long way from cancer when you have cervical dysplasia, and cervical cancer is one of the slowest-growing cancers. In other words, unless you have a Class IV or Class V pap smear, it is rarely a reason to panic or rush into surgery. Take the time to get another pap smear from a different laboratory, as well as a second opinion from another doctor. Nearly six out of eight times, the second pap smear will come out negative.

A common cause of cervical dysplasia is a viral infection of cervical cells caused by human papillomavirus (HPV), a sexually transmitted disease that causes condyloma warts or lesions in the genital area and the cervix.

When you have a Class II pap smear and genital warts, your physician may want to do an actual biopsy because some of the HPV viral subtypes are more likely to be cancerous or potentially cancerous, and some are completely without the potential to be malignant.

When cervical dysplasia is found, it is important to ask yourself why your body hasn't protected you from HPV and inflammation. Many things can irritate and inflame the cervix and cause a Class II pap smear, including traumatic or unloving sex, tampons, condoms, douches, and spermicide (found on condoms and used with diaphragms and cervical caps). Progesterone deficiency also contributes to dysplasia and may make the cervix more susceptible to the above irritations.

Cervicitis (infection or inflammation of the cervix), a chlamydia infection, and sexual trauma can all temporarily look like cervical dysplasia. Smoking increases a woman's chances of cervical irritation and, eventually, dysplasia. Dr. Hanley has found that when a woman is having sexual intercourse that is not really friendly to her and her body, and she is not saying no because she wants so much to please her mate, it is physically traumatizing to her body and especially to her cervix. Sometimes the end of a man's penis will run into a woman's cervix and cause physical trauma. All of this can show up initially as an abnormal Class II or III pap smear. If it's clear that the cellular abnormality showing up on a pap smear is not a viral infection or a cancer, the most sensible suggestion is to return in three to six months for another one. Women who get repeated cervical infections such as chlamydia should make sure their partner isn't reinfecting them.

When Dr. Hanley sees a woman with a Class II pap smear, she most often suggests that she use an aloe vera or acidophilus douche or suppositories for a few weeks, along with taking folic acid (5 to 10 mg daily), vitamin A (10,000 IU daily), vitamin B6 (25 to 50 mg daily) and vitamin B12, 800 to 1,000 mcg. She also recommends vitamin A oil put directly onto the cervix five out of seven nights per week for four weeks, two weeks off, and then for four more weeks. You can buy vitamin A suppositories, break open capsules, or use a liquid vitamin A with a dropper. Dr. Hanley recommends that with the high doses of folic acid used in this type of treatment (a normal dose is 400 mcg), women work in partnership with a health care professional.

Dr. Lee's daughter was told she needed a cervical cone biopsy, a major surgery, and her father encouraged her to first try using some progesterone, 400 mcg daily of folic acid, and 50 mg daily of vitamin B6. Sure enough, within three cycles her dysplasia was gone.

If it looks like an infection is present, Dr. Hanley may suggest a hydrogen peroxide douche consisting of a ¼ cup of hydrogen peroxide and 2 cups of water for a couple of nights before bed. Another option is a goldenseal douche, which she has found will get rid of most organisms within a couple of days of use.

❧ CERVICAL DYSPLASIA AND HORMONES

Cervical dysplasia was relatively rare before the advent of oral contraceptives. We now know that oral contraceptives increase the risk of cervical dysplasia by at least 50 percent and the risk of cervical cancer by at least 25 percent. In a 1994 study done by Dr. Giske Ursin of the University of Southern California and published in the medical journal *Lancet,* researchers found that being on birth control pills for only one to six months increased the risk of cervical cancer three times. Ursin believes the study explains why the incidence of cervical cancer more than doubled in the United States between the early 1970s and the mid-1980s, which parallels the advent of widespread use of oral contraceptives.

Part of the dynamic of this, in addition to excessive exposure to estrogen and deficiency of real progesterone, may be that birth control pills deplete the B vitamins, especially folic acid, which can be a direct cause of cervical dysplasia. Bottom line: If you must take oral contraceptives (or shots or implants) and you have an abnormal pap smear, you should stop taking them.

Clearly the long-term health benefits of avoiding birth control pills outweigh the inconvenience caused by other methods of birth control. You can refer to chapter 11 for more information about birth control.

Doctors have become careless about prescribing estrogen and are beginning to prescribe unopposed estrogen to premenopausal women with hormonal symptoms. Giving a premenopausal woman unopposed estrogen is almost the same as writing a prescription for cervical dysplasia—she will almost certainly return to the doctor's office within a year and have a positive pap smear. The next step is then a hysterectomy, followed by a prescription for Premarin and Provera. You absolutely do not need to go that route.

When Dr. Hanley sees a woman with a Class III pap smear who is opposed to surgery (or who prefers to give alternative treatments a try first), the first thing she does is ask the woman to take a close look at her sexual relationship with her partner and to make some dietary changes, with particular attention paid to avoiding dairy foods. (More details on diet are available in chapter 14.) In addition to the supplements recommended above, Dr. Hanley also adds 30 mg of zinc daily, 500 mg of vitamin C daily, an antioxidant mix, and a multivitamin.

Since a Class III cervical dysplasia can be caused or aggravated by the excessive cell proliferation caused by estrogen dominance, she often recommends the use of progesterone cream to oppose the estrogen effects, along with the vitamins mentioned above. Women sometimes ask if they can put the progesterone directly onto the cervix. Although it isn't necessary, it is fine to do if you're very sure it's a pure progesterone cream that contains no carcinogenic chemical preservatives and no estrogenic herbs. To use it that way, look for a cream that contains only progesterone as its active ingredient.

It's very common for a doctor to recommend that a woman with a Class II pap smear have a surgery called a conization, or cone biopsy, in which a circle of tissue around the inside of the cervix is removed with a knife or a laser. This is a major surgery that involves general anesthesia. Continued bleeding and infection are common complications, and fertility is frequently affected by interfering with the production of cervical mucus. A cone biopsy may also result in miscarriages because the cervix is unable to stay closed. Using a laser in this procedure may sound more high tech, but the results can be equally destructive.

❧ HEALING THE CERVIX ❧

What to Do for Cervical Dysplasia

- Use an aloe vera and/or acidophilus douche before bed.
- Take folic acid, 400 mcg daily, or 5–10 mg daily working with a health care professional.
- Take vitamin B6, 25–50 mg daily.
- Take vitamin B12, 800–1,000 mcg daily.
- Take vitamin A, 10,000 IU orally daily and topically on the cervix.
- Take vitamin E, 400 IU daily.
- Use natural progesterone cream.*

What to Do for Cervical Inflammation and Infection

- Douche with ¼ cup hydrogen peroxide to 2 cups water before bed two nights in a row.

- Take vitamin A, 10,000 IU daily (orally and/or rub directly on the cervix).

What to Avoid

- Unopposed estrogen
- Birth control pills
- Spermicides (used in diaphragm jelly and on condoms)
- Commercial douches
- Tampons
- Unloving, unwanted, or traumatic sex

*See chapter 16 for details on how to use natural progesterone cream.

Chapter 7

❖

Cycles, Follicles, and Ovaries

Amanda was having pelvic pain in the middle of her menstrual cycle and severe bloating premenstrually, and had developed chronic headaches. During a pelvic exam, her ob-gyn could feel an enlarged ovary, and an ultrasound showed that she had a large ovarian cyst on her right ovary. Because some types of ovarian cyst can become cancerous, and blood tests are inconclusive, her doctor wanted to do exploratory surgery to rule out cancer. Amanda arrived in Dr. Hanley's office clutching her abdomen and declaring, "I don't want them to take my ovaries!"

Dr. Hanley read Amanda's ob-gyn report, asked her detailed questions about her family health history and lifestyle, and suggested an AMAS (which stands for anti-malignan antibody in serum) test. The AMAS test is a remarkable and revolutionary test that can detect, with an extremely high accuracy rate, even a microscopic malignant cancer anywhere in the body. You can read chapter 12 to learn more, and you can find out how and where to get one in the Resources section in the back of the book.

Amanda had no family history of ovarian cancer; she seemed to be a little bit androgen (male hormone) dominant; and she was pushing herself extremely hard to keep up with a job and a boss she didn't like, three small children, and a difficult relationship with her ex-husband. Dr. Hanley felt that once an AMAS test ruled out the existence of a malignant ovarian cancer (which it did), Amanda would have the opportunity to freely work with herself to bring her body into balance rather than rushing into a surgery for an ovarian cyst that might or might not be cancerous.

Amanda was a creative and artistically gifted woman who found herself working every day in an office management position to support her children. Although she considered raising her children to be very creative, and often worked with them on art projects, she craved the time and solitude to create her own art projects. She felt trapped in her job and stifled artistically. Dr. Hanley suggested that Amanda use her creative powers to find a small space in her home and a few hours a week for her own art. Amanda commandeered a corner in the laundry room and set up an area where she could do clay sculptures in the early morning hours. As she sculpted, she began to have ideas about how she could create a better position for herself within her company and get out from under her domineering boss.

Dr. Hanley also worked with Amanda to create a more balanced diet, which had been heavy on the pizza, bagels, and dairy products, and gave her some herbs and supplements to help maintain her blood sugar balance and support her liver. She encouraged Amanda to write or draw in a journal at least a few times a week and to find activities with the kids that included exercise.

Making positive changes in her life was difficult for someone as busy and driven as Amanda, but as she took small steps in the right direction, she was rewarded with fewer headaches and less bloating premenstrually. After three months she was making good progress, and her symptoms, though not completely gone, were significantly reduced. She had another ultrasound, which showed that her ovarian cyst was less than half the size it had been, and another AMAS test, which was negative. She decided to continue working with Dr. Hanley rather than having surgery.

A year later, Amanda was having some cycles with minor symptoms of pain, bloating, and headaches and some cycles that were symptom-free, and through paying attention to herself and keeping a journal of symptoms, she felt she had learned to keep her body's tendency to form ovarian cysts in balance. She had discovered a very strong correlation between her symptoms and not taking good care of herself, and that became a great motivation to stay on track.

❧ HANG ON TO YOUR OVARIES IF YOU CAN

Your ovaries are the anatomical equivalent of a man's testicles, and just as the testicles in a man are a source of hormone-generated energy and libido, your ovaries serve a similar function. And just as removing a man's testicles is castration, removing your ovaries is castration. No kidding! That is the medical term for removing a woman's ovaries, and that's exactly what it is, with all the implications that go with that loaded word. The effect of castration can be just as profound in a woman as in a man, although your doctor is likely to be adamant that it will solve all your problems. It's possible that your doctor is correct, in the same sense that castrating a man will solve all of his "problems."

Once a man is castrated and he no longer makes any appreciable amounts of testosterone, he will be less aggressive, will have little or no libido, will gain some weight, and will begin to develop osteoporosis within a year or two. A woman who is castrated and no longer makes any appreciable amounts of estrogen, progesterone, and androstenedione will often become depressed, have little to no libido, and, with the addition of some Premarin, she will be retaining water and will probably be anxious as well. She will also have an increased risk of osteoporosis and heart disease, even if she takes replacement hormones. If she is put just on Premarin, which most women without a uterus are (assuming that if her ovaries are removed her uterus will also be removed), her risk of breast cancer will rise, especially after five years. She will lose the small amounts of hormones her ovaries would have been making, even menopausally, putting all of the burden and additional stress on her adrenal glands to produce the needed steroid hormones. Even if she supplements with all of the steroid hormones, they will not be as well regulated as they would have been by her ovaries.

There are relatively rare instances when it's wise and appropriate to have your ovaries removed. The most obvious is ovarian cancer. Other reasons to remove the ovaries include ovarian cysts that have a high risk of being precancerous, and extremely enlarged ovarian cysts that are causing pain and don't respond to treatment. But the vast majority of these surgeries, called oophorectomies, are unnecessary.

One reason doctors tend to be eager to remove your ovaries is that they are afraid of ovarian cancer and see oophorectomy as preventive medicine. Even though ovarian cancer is relatively rare, it is very scary to those who have seen someone go through it, because it is difficult to diagnose until it is fairly advanced, and it has a very low rate of remission in conventional medicine. If a doctor views ovaries as useless after the reproductive years and ovarian cancer as a frightening disease, you can understand why he or she would be anxious to remove them. What your doctor may not realize is that even after removing the ovaries, cancer can appear in the pelvic cavity that behaves just like ovarian cancer. What this means to you is that prevention is important, especially if there are women in your immediate family who have had ovarian cancer. Your risk of ovarian cancer increases if you have used fertility drugs such as Clomid, if you have used birth control pills, or if you have been ovulating for as long as you have been menstruating (i.e., you haven't been pregnant). Preventing cancer is discussed in detail in chapters 12 and 14.

❧ A LITTLE BIT ON WHAT WE KNOW ABOUT YOUR OVARIES

You would probably be astounded at how much medical science *doesn't* know about the inner workings of your ovaries and how the ovaries are stimulated to produce and release hormones. We do, however, know enough to give you some basic information on keeping your ovaries and keeping them healthy.

When your menstrual cycles are regular and functioning optimally, your ovaries release an egg into the fallopian tube every eighteen to twenty-eight days. The release of the egg is called ovulation (see figures 7.1 and 7.2). But let's back up a moment to find out what takes place before the egg is released from the ovary.

When an egg in residence in the ovary responds to hormonal signals from the brain, the tissue surrounding it begins to enlarge and matures into a follicle, which moves to the outside edge of the ovary. As it enlarges, the follicle begins to make estrogens. Every month about 120 follicles are enlisted in the process of maturing eggs, but normally only one succeeds in releasing the egg (ovu-

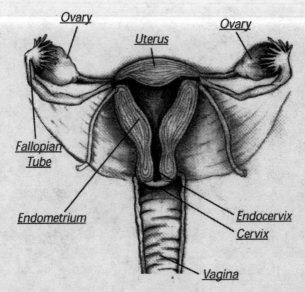

Figure 7.1. Front View of Reproductive System

lation) before the others. With ovulation, the follicle becomes the corpus luteum and makes abundant progesterone, which stops further ovulation by the rest of the follicles as well as the follicles of the other ovary.

When the egg is released from the follicle, it doesn't just fall into the fallopian tube; it is some distance away (relatively speaking) and is drawn there (by what, we don't know exactly). Dr. Lee had a patient who had no ovary on her right side and no fallopian tube on her left side. When she remarried in her early forties she assumed

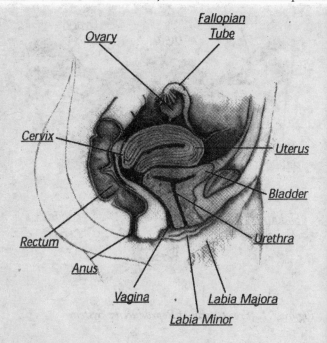

Figure 7.2. Side View of Reproductive System

she was infertile but, lo and behold, she became pregnant. Somehow an egg from the remaining ovary had found its way to the remaining fallopian tube on the opposite side of the body and migrated to the uterus. Nine months later she gave birth to a healthy baby boy.

❧ WHAT AGES FIRST, THE OVARY OR THE BRAIN?

There is a chicken-and-egg argument among researchers who study the biochemistry of aging, about whether menopause happens when the hormonal signals from the brain that stimulate the maturation of the follicle begin to fail or whether it is the ovary and its follicles that fail to respond to the signals from the brain. We'll probably find that it is both, with predispositions caused by genetically inherited and environmental effects.

Based on the people she sees every day in her office, Dr. Hanley believes that environmental estrogens, called xenoestrogens or xenohormones, are elevated to the point that they are suppressing our LH (luteinizing hormone), which is the pituitary hormone that signals the ovaries to release the egg and to make progesterone. She consistently sees lower-than-normal LH levels in women in their forties. She has noticed that the women she sees with low LH levels have a difficult time getting pregnant, and they are more prone to have PMS, irregular bleeding, and abnormal menstrual cycles. She theorizes that though the ovaries are capable of manufacturing the hormones, they aren't receiving enough stimulus from the brain to do the job.

If you don't ovulate in any given month (called an anovulatory cycle) you will release little to no progesterone, because it is the empty follicle, now called the corpus luteum, that is primarily responsible for manufacturing your monthly surges of progesterone. Imagine the delicacy of your hormonal balance, when the release of one microscopic egg plays a leading role in maintaining it.

During your entire life span, you only have about ten to fifteen years, from your early twenties to your mid-thirties, when you ovulate pretty much every month. Before puberty you do not ovulate, through puberty you will ovulate some months and not others, and as you reach premenopausal age, ovulation will begin to be irregular again. Women who are doing heavy physical exercise, who are on extremely low-calorie (or very low-fat) diets, who are under heavy stress, or who are ill, will often not ovulate. Any month that you don't ovulate, you are more susceptible to hormonal imbalances, particularly estrogen dominance.

Even when you don't ovulate and produce the corresponding surge of progesterone, if your estrogen levels are sufficient to build up the blood-rich lining of your uterus, you will have a menstrual cycle when your estrogen levels fall at the end of the month. In other words, just because you are menstruating doesn't mean that you are ovulating. Menstrual cycles do not depend completely on progesterone, although they tend to be more regular and free of symptoms when progesterone is present, either through ovulation or supplementation.

Sometimes ovulation will occur, but the follicle is dysfunctional and progesterone production will fade earlier than normal in the cycle. When that happens, estrogen dominance recurs during the weeks before menstruation despite ovulation. And in such a case, even if fertilization occurs, the human chorionic gonadotropin (HCG) signal from the fertilized egg may not result in sufficient progesterone for successful implantation and the pregnancy fails without the woman ever being aware of it.

❖ YOUR OVARIES ARE WORKING FOR YOU FOR A LIFETIME

Contrary to the myth popular among conventional medical doctors, your ovaries do not entirely shut down when you stop having menstrual cycles. Like most glands, your ovary is a complex structure with a multitude of functions. The thin outer layer, called the theca, produces eggs. That layer becomes increasingly nonfunctional as you age. The inner layer, called the ovarian stroma, is capable of manufacturing all of the steroid hormones, and there is increasing evidence that it functions to some extent throughout your life. Overall, your hormone levels will naturally decline with age (see figure 1.1). Around menopause, the stroma begins to produce more androstenedione, a male hormone, that can be converted to estrogen in the fat cells as needed. Women who develop symptoms of androgen dominance such as thinning hair on the head, heavier hair growth above the lip, and a prominent belly may be lacking in the enzymes or enzyme cofactors (usually vitamins and minerals) necessary to convert androstenedione to estrogen.

Biochemist David Zava's research shows that insulin resistance, resulting in high levels of insulin in the blood, plays a primary role in blocking the conversion of androstenedione to estrogen and also directly blocks the pathways through which estrogen and other hormones are synthesized. Insulin resistance is most often caused by obesity.

❧ YOUR OVARIES HAVE MANY FORMS OF EXPRESSION

When a woman complains of chronic pelvic pain and enlarged ovarian cysts show up on an ultrasound, they are often used as a justification for removing the ovaries. It's important that you know that most of the time the presence of cysts on the ovary is completely normal and that enlarged cysts are common and are rarely cancerous.

Cysts are a normal part of the ovulatory process. Prior to ovulation, anywhere from a few to a few hundred follicles will mature and enlarge in the ovary enough to become cyst-like. Normally only one follicle will release its egg into the fallopian tube, leaving the others to go through various forms and stages of reabsorption into the ovary or dissolution outside of the ovary.

When a number of follicles migrate to the surface of the ovary, but none releases egg, no progesterone is made. The hypothalamus is monitoring for both estrogen and progesterone levels. When progesterone fails to rise, the hypothalamus signals the pituitary (by releasing a substance called gonadotropin-releasing hormone or GnRH) to make more follicle stimulating hormone (FSH). FSH tells the ovary to get back to the work of maturing an egg. The increased FSH results in only more estrogen production. The follicles become cysts that are stimulated to grow even larger with each succeeding cycle. Some ovarian cysts burst into the pelvic cavity, releasing blood and fluid, which can cause pain. When progesterone levels are restored to normal for a few months the cysts are usually uneventfully reabsorbed.

There is an amazing amount of variation in ovarian cysts, normal and abnormal. They can spring up almost overnight, and they can go away just as fast. They can grow to be as big as a lemon or even larger before they disappear. If a cyst is over four centimeters, your doctor will probably tell you it is abnormal and should be removed. A more rational and conservative option is to watch the cyst for a few months and see if it goes away, which it most often does.

Some cysts are fluid filled, and some become more solid. In general, the more solid an ovarian cyst is at the core, the greater its chance of becoming cancerous. For reasons not clear, it sometimes happens that ovaries contain a follicle with the ability to make skin cells, teeth, hair, or other tissue. When such a follicle is stimulated by FSH, some of these tissues may develop within a cyst. These rare dermoid cysts are not reabsorbed, they grow monthly, and need to be removed surgically.

Women with high estrogen and low progesterone levels, and women with high androgen levels, may have polycystic (many cysts) ovaries, in which many small, undeveloped follicles remain just under the outer covering of the ovary, making it large and lumpy.

❖ THE EMOTIONAL SIDE OF
   YOUR OVARIES

When Dr. Hanley works with a woman who has an ovarian cyst, she always asks what traumatic event recently took place in her life. She finds that, particularly with premenopausal women, life's traumas and disruptions are often reflected in the ovaries and that an emotionally challenging or frightening event at the right time in the cycle is enough to throw the hormonal orchestra into temporary or even chronic chaos.

As a woman enters her forties, she is more likely to grow what's called a functional ovarian cyst, which is created because her hormones are not orchestrating perfectly and the egg is never released from the follicle. This kind of cyst may go completely unnoticed or may cause discomfort and become chronic. Some of the symptoms may be irregular breathing; periods that are too early, too heavy, or too light; or pain on one side of the pelvis or abdomen that can range from a small pinch to severe stabbing pain.

The symptoms are often preceded by a dramatic life event, although it doesn't have to be a completely emotional trauma. Traveling across the continent or an ocean is enough to do it. More often, however, Dr. Hanley discovers the woman with the ovarian cyst has had a husband or boyfriend who was unfaithful or walked out, or who got bad news about her child's health, or who had sudden financial problems. Defusing the emotions around such an event by confiding in a friend or family member, getting counseling, or writing in a journal, can work wonders to prevent and heal functional ovarian cysts.

Dr. Hanley also finds that when the traumatic event is connected to anger or rage at another person, or even at ourselves when we've been in denial about our problems, working with forgiveness is powerfully healing. We do not forgive other people for their sake; we forgive them for our sake. It is the only truly effective way to let go of hurt, anger, and rage so that we don't keep recreating it in our bodies.

❖ MAKING ESTROGEN AFTER MENOPAUSE

Next time you're out and about, observe the women around you. You'll see that the vast majority of women between the ages of forty and seventy are a little bit plump. You'll see this almost anywhere in the world that you travel. Estrogen production in fat cells may be nature's reason for putting weight on women around the time of menopause: As your ovarian production of estrogen falls, your fat cells will pick up some of the slack. In spite of our intense cultural conditioning to the contrary, a little bit of plumpness (not obesity) in women around the menopausal years is probably a very beneficial and important protective mechanism designed to promote the production of estrogen in the fat cells, which plays a role in preventing bone loss and keeping the brain active.

Women who are heavier at menopause tend to have

higher estrogen levels, fewer "menopausal" symptoms, and less osteoporosis. But they do also have a higher risk of breast cancer. As always, there's a balance here. Excessive weight gain is unhealthy and causes myriad hormone and other imbalances. Heavy women who have hot flashes are almost always those who are obese, have had their ovaries removed, and/or who smoke.

Around the age of seventy, women tend to start becoming thin again. Ovarian function may have wound down so much at that age that even androstenedione production is low. But even with such low hormone production, women who are relatively healthy at that age tend to have the keen interest in life that they had when they were preadolescents, combined with the wisdom and humor that comes with having lived seven decades on earth.

❧ INCREASING YOUR AWARENESS OF YOUR OVARIES

Your ovaries are very active glands. Many women can feel it when they ovulate; they say it feels like a pinching or slight cramping sensation in the area of the ovary, which is below and to either side of the navel. It could easily be mistaken for a case of gas or indigestion. Becoming aware of when you ovulate is a wonderful way to become more aware of your body and its cycles.

Awareness of your ovaries will also give you fertility awareness. You'll find that when you ovulate your vaginal mucus will change, first becoming more profuse or "wet," and then also becoming more clear, slippery, and stretchy, almost like raw egg whites.

One of the ways to tell if you are ovulating is to take your temperature under your armpit as soon as you wake up in the morning, starting on the last day of your menstrual period. You'll find that when you ovulate your temperature will go up as much as one degree.

You can also buy a device that is essentially a minimicroscope and look at your vaginal mucus. When you ovulate your vaginal mucus will create a distinct ferning pattern that you can easily see. When you aren't ovulating the mucus will appear normal. (See the Resources section.)

Strictly speaking, you are only fertile for about seventy-two hours each cycle. Considering that sperm may live up to seventy-two hours after being inseminated into the vagina, it is theoretically possible that conception can occur from sperm arriving two to three days prior to actual ovulation. Thus, the opportunity for conception may extend over a six-day period each month. Women who are aware of their ovulation through the methods described above can use that as a form of birth control, which is 98 percent effective when used conscientiously.

As a premenopausal woman who is not necessarily ovulating every month, you can also use your awareness to know when you are not ovulating. Some premenopausal women only use progesterone cream during the months that they know they haven't ovulated because that's the only time they need it. This is a beautiful and balanced use of body awareness and conscious hormone balancing. Not every woman is that tuned in, but if you are, use it to your advantage with your hormone balance program.

We hope that as women begin to value their reproductive organs, including their ovaries, physicians will follow their lead. Throughout your life, your ovaries are a precious source of energy and hormone production that works in much greater harmony with the rest of your body than any hormone replacement program ever could.

❖ HEALING THE OVARIES ❖

What to Do

- If estrogen-dominance symptoms are present, use some natural progesterone cream.*
- For functional ovarian cysts, take a liver-supporting and detoxifying herbal formula that includes some or all of the following herbs: *Bupleurum,* milk thistle (*Silybum marianum*), barberry or goldenseal, burdock root, yellow dock, dandelion root.
- For functional ovarian cysts, take an ovary-healing herbal formula that includes some or all of the following herbs: burdock root, cramp bark (*Viburnum opulus*), licorice root, dandelion root, *Vitex,* red raspberry.
- Take a good multivitamin-mineral daily.

What to Do to Restore Ovulation

- Manage stress more effectively and slow down.
- Avoid very strenuous exercise.
- Avoid very low calorie diets.
- Take the herb *Vitex* (follow directions on the container).
- Use some natural progesterone cream on days 5–26 for three cycles to temporarily suppress ovulation. On the fourth cycle, ovulation will often occur.
- Work through traumatic events with creative outlets, therapy, journal writing, and so on.
- Leave abusive relationships.

What to Avoid

- Unopposed estrogen and estrogen dominance
- Birth control pills
- Fertility drugs
- Talcum powder in the genital area
- Dairy products
- Feed-lot meats (eat only range-fed organic meats free of drugs and pesticide residues)

*See chapter 16 for details on how to use natural progesterone cream.

Chapter 8

❧

PMS: And When She Was Good She Was Very, Very Good, and When She Was Bad She Was Horrid

*P*remenstrual syndrome or PMS is by far the single most common complaint of premenopausal women. Current estimates are that severe PMS occurs in 2.5 to 5 percent of women, and mild PMS occurs in 33 percent of women. PMS was first described in 1931 as a "state of unbearable tension," a description most women can understand to a certain degree. Some women have PMS from the time they begin having menstrual cycles but for most, PMS begins in the premenopausal years, around the mid-thirties, and becomes increasingly severe as the years go on. Although it's possible to create a list of dozens and dozens of PMS symptoms, the most common are bloating and water retention (and the resulting weight gain), breast tenderness and lumpiness, headaches, cramps, fatigue, irritability, mood swings, and anxiety. In women with severe PMS, irritability and mood swings can become outbursts of anger and rage. By definition, PMS symptoms occur in the two weeks before menstruation and sometimes for a few days into menstruation.

You should know right up front that there is no "magic bullet" for PMS. A little bit of progesterone will help a lot, and in some women it solves the problem, because it offsets the effects of environmental estrogens and anovulatory cycles. But PMS is a multifactorial problem that needs to be handled on many physical levels as well as on the emotional level. You'll discover more about the emotional level when we talk about the emotional side of premenopause later in the chapter.

Stress is almost always involved in PMS. Stress increases levels of cortisol, which blocks progesterone from its receptors. Therefore, normal progesterone levels do *not* mean that supplemental progesterone is not needed. Extra progesterone is necessary to overcome the blockade of its receptors by cortisol. When a woman discovers she has a handle on controlling her PMS, it will help her manage stress better. Then lower levels of progesterone will work normally again.

For years it was assumed that since PMS symptoms occur when progesterone levels are normally relatively high, it was progesterone that was causing the symptoms. Theoretically, symptoms could relate either to elevated progesterone levels or progesterone deficiency (estrogen dominance). Elevated levels of progesterone are unlikely since, during pregnancy, progesterone levels are ten to twenty times higher than normal midcycle levels and similar symptoms do not occur. Progesterone deficiency (estrogen dominance) is more likely since many of the symptoms correlate with estrogen-dominance symptoms, most notably water retention, breast swelling, headaches, mood swings, loss of libido, and poor sleep patterns.

A woman's response to her own cyclical hormones is extremely individual, and this is part of the reason that it has been so difficult to pin down the causes of PMS. Estrogen levels that cause anxiety and bloating in one woman will have virtually no effect on another. A woman who sails through an anovulatory cycle with hardly a ripple offers a complete contrast to the woman who is plagued by migraines or anger premenstrually when she doesn't ovulate. Birth control pills and premenopausal hormone replacement therapy (HRT) will cause a long list of side effects (including PMS) in many women, whereas others will say they feel fine. This is why it's so important that you become familiar with your own body and your own symptoms, and don't let anybody tell you that what you're experiencing is "just an emotional problem" or that an antidepressant or tranquilizer is all you need.

The first attempts at using progesterone to treat PMS symptoms were only partially successful. High-dose vaginal or rectal progesterone suppositories, pioneered by the British researcher Katherina Dalton, M.D., had some success, but the results weren't consistent. Now we know that using high doses of progesterone leads to the formation of metabolites (excretion by-products) in the liver that are not progesterone, that inhibit progesterone at receptor sites, and that can cause undesirable side effects or block the effects of the progesterone. Oral progesterone (pill form), which is given in high doses of 100 to 300 mg, may have the same unfortunate effect. (Oral progesterone must be prescribed in very high doses because the liver immediately dumps up to 90 percent of it.)

Even with the limitations and drawbacks of the high doses needed in oral progesterone, Dr. Joel T. Hargrove of Vanderbilt University Medical Center, has published results indicating a 90 percent success rate in treating PMS with oral doses of natural micronized progesterone.

An article recently published by Peter J. Schmidt in the *New England Journal of Medicine*, studied women who were given a drug (Lupron) that suppresses ovarian hormones altogether. Some of the women who had PMS reported that their symptoms were significantly better when they took the drug. Schmidt and his colleagues took that group of women and gave them either Lupron plus transdermal estradiol, or Lupron plus 200 mg progesterone twice daily in the form of vaginal suppositories, both for ten weeks.

The idea was that with the body's natural hormones suppressed, the women would be exposed to either one or the other hormone, and whichever one caused symptoms would be the PMS culprit. This completely ignores the fact that steroid hormones depend on a delicate balance and orchestration of all of them, and the constant ten-week suppression and exposure ignores the cyclical nature of hormones. On top of that, the massive doses of 400 mg progesterone daily is enough to throw any woman's body into hormonal chaos.

Both the estradiol and the progesterone groups reported that their PMS symptoms returned. Considering the inappropriately huge dose of progesterone, plus the fact that when first given progesterone tends to stimulate estrogen receptors for one or two cycles, this result is not surprising. Had they given the women transdermal progesterone in appropriate two-week cycles for three months, which is enough time to allow progesterone's activation of estrogen receptors to subside, they would have found that the women on progesterone improved greatly.

As it was, the researchers expressed surprise that estrogen caused PMS symptoms. Their conclusion was that "in women with premenstrual syndrome, the occurrence of symptoms represents an abnormal response to normal hormonal changes." Rather than call women who are sensitive to hormonal fluctuations "abnormal," it is more accurate to say that women differ greatly in their response to hormonal fluctuations and imbalances and that some women are more sensitive to hormones than others. However, since the study was a poorly disguised attempt to promote the drug Lupron to treat PMS, it benefits the makers of Lupron to declare that women who are sensitive to hormonal changes are "abnormal." Don't you believe it!

The other typical mistake made by doctors trying to

treat PMS with progesterone is thinking that the synthetic progestins are the same as progesterone. Giving progestins to a woman with PMS is like throwing gasoline on a fire—for most women it will only make symptoms dramatically worse.

Progesterone cream used in normal doses of 15 to 30 mg daily for two weeks a month has a very high success rate in relieving PMS symptoms. According to Dr. Hanley, some women who are very deficient may need to use up to 100 mg twice a day for a month or two, and then gradually reduce their dose. Dr. Lee has letters from hundreds of women telling him how their PMS disappeared when they used progesterone cream. He has noticed that women whose PMS symptoms include edema (swelling, bloating, water retention, weight gain) experience the most relief. (The details on how to use progesterone to treat PMS are found in chapter 16.)

Margaret Smith, M.D., a highly regarded hormone researcher and clinician from Australia, reported in a recent talk that progesterone cream is the most effective treatment for PMS that she has yet to observe. She also noted that a colleague of hers recorded hormone levels in 50 women for over 20 years, and he found that PMS consistently correlated with low progesterone levels and high estrogen levels.

Dr. Hanley uses progesterone cream as the core of her PMS treatment program, but especially in younger women her goal is to create enough balance within the whole woman so that progesterone is needed only occasionally. In women of any age, just using progesterone cream often completely eliminates PMS. Combining progesterone with stress management and diet is the most successful strategy.

The most important physical influences on PMS are hormonal imbalances caused by stress, diet, and environmental toxins. There is also a very real and very natural increase in sensitivity in a woman premenstrually, which is too often condemned and misunderstood. That aspect of PMS will be covered in detail in the section in this chapter on the emotional side of PMS.

❧ PMS AND THE STRESS CONNECTION

You know from chapter 2 that stress increases your levels of cortisol, a hormone released primarily by the adrenal glands in response to feelings of fear, danger, or even a sense of competition. In excess, cortisol can stimulate feelings of irritability, anger, and rage. Cortisol is also released when you push yourself to work through tiredness day after day. Think of cortisol as a backup energy system. Like the batteries that back up your electronics when the electrical power goes out, you can't just keep using them to give you full power, or they'll wear out and you'll also lose that source of energy. In the same way, you can't depend on your cortisol and your adrenal glands to keep taking you beyond your physical limits or eventually you will create depleted organs and chronic fatigue.

Since cortisol and progesterone compete for common receptors in the cells, cortisol impairs progesterone activity, setting the stage for estrogen dominance. Chronically elevated cortisol levels can be a direct cause of estrogen dominance, with all the familiar PMS symptoms.

High cortisol levels also affect blood sugar. Cortisol sends glucose (blood sugar) flooding into the cells. The initial rush of glucose into the cells may feel great, but twenty or so minutes later your body will be working overtime to find more glucose, and you'll be searching the cupboards or your desk drawers for candy bars, cookies, and potato chips to get your blood sugar and your energy back up. The majority of those empty calories will be converted to fat, and if you keep up the pattern long term, you'll be struggling to keep your weight down and your energy up.

Fluctuating blood sugar creates another type of negative feedback cycle, where high levels of sugar in the blood stimulate the release of adrenaline, which in turn stimulates the release of cortisol, which in turn causes a craving for quick calories, and so forth.

Stress also raises levels of a hormone called prolactin, which is best known as the hormone that stimulates the breasts to make milk. High levels of prolactin reduce progesterone production, which in turn stimulates higher prolactin levels. A good example of the prolactin-progesterone feedback loop is a woman in her last trimester of pregnancy who makes some 300 mg of progesterone a day through the placenta. At birth, the abrupt drop in progesterone signals the body to raise prolactin levels, which stimulates milk production in the breasts. Thus high prolactin levels suppress progesterone, and low progesterone levels can in turn stimulate prolactin synthesis.

Other factors that can raise prolactin levels include hypothyroidism (low thyroid); herpes zoster; estrogens; oral contraceptives; and a number of prescription drugs, including L-dopa, reserpine, the phenothiazines (antipsychotic drugs), the tricyclic antidepressants, and, to a lesser extent, the antiulcer drug metoclopramide (Reglan) and the over-the-counter H_2 (histamine) blockers used to treat heartburn such as cimetidine (Tagamet) and ranitidine (Zantac).

Elevated prolactin levels and prolactinomas (prolactin-producing tumors of the pituitary) are becoming increasingly common. In fact, prolactinomas are now the number-one intracranial (brain) tumor. If found, a trial of progesterone supplementation is recommended, since progesterone will inhibit the release of prolactin by the pituitary.

The effect of raised prolactin levels in depressing progesterone isn't as dramatic as cortisol, but it's another factor in the hormonal imbalance profile of PMS that should be taken into account when considering the whole picture.

You can give your body all the progesterone it needs, but if it's still competing with cortisol and prolactin—in other words, if you don't manage the stress in your life more effectively—you'll still be running at least partially on your back-up energy systems. Progesterone can provide a partial antidote to high cortisol and prolactin levels and the resulting PMS symptoms, but ultimately you need to bring your cortisol back to normal.

❧ PMS AND THE ESSENTIAL FATTY ACIDS

Prostaglandins are hormone-like substances that regulate every cell in the body in a multilevel series of complex interactions. Although the tendency in medicine is to identify "good" and "bad" prostaglandins, in truth they are all needed for balance, and it is an imbalance of prostaglandins that can promote heart disease, immune system dysfunction, inflammation, pain, and PMS. One of the reasons that aspirin is such a popular drug is that it very effectively blocks all prostaglandins and in the process dramatically reduces inflammation. This makes aspirin good medicine for a short-term problem like a headache, but over the long run, you don't want to be suppressing your entire prostaglandin system. This is one of the big drawbacks of the common recommendation of conventional medical doctors to take an aspirin every day to prevent a heart attack.

When prostaglandins are out of balance, your blood is more likely to clump together, raising your risk of a stroke or heart attack. Since estrogen dominance has the same effect on the blood, the combination of imbalanced prostaglandins and estrogen effects can create more severe symptoms. Supplements such as evening primrose oil and borage oil contain high levels of gamma-linolenic acid (GLA) oils that stimulate the anti-inflammatory prostaglandins and can help ease PMS symptoms.

One of the easiest ways to get your prostaglandins out of balance and create chronic inflammation is to eat foods that contain hydrogenated oils (trans-fatty acids) found in margarines and in most cakes, cookies, and chips, which show up on labels as "partially hydrogenated." These synthetic oils block the effect of the natural oils, which have important and potent regulatory effects on your prostaglandins. Eating the rancid vegetable oils found in these processed foods when they *aren't* hydrogenated also creates prostaglandin imbalances.

Other causes of imbalanced prostaglandins are too much sugar in the diet, viral illnesses such as herpes, and—you guessed it—stress. The release of stress hormones stimulates the inflammation-producing prostaglandins, which may be good news if you're injured or fighting off an illness but causes chronic problems such as PMS when it is a daily occurrence. Inflammation raises both cortisol and estrogen levels, and it suppresses progesterone.

It is also possible that zinc deficiency contributes to essential fatty acid (EFA) imbalances, since zinc, vitamin C, and some of the B vitamins are needed to make the conversion from an unsaturated oil to the needed EFAs.

Nutritional fads come and go with great regularity, and it is currently nutritionally faddish to take supplements containing large amounts of the so-called "good" oils such as those found in borage oil, evening primrose oil, and flax seed oil. These oils, along with pumpkin and walnut oils, can be very useful for treating inflammation-related symptoms such as PMS or a headache in the short term, in much the same way that aspirin is useful. But normally we only need the EFAs in the tiny amounts found in fresh fruits, raw nuts, vegetables, and whole grains. In the category of the EFAs known as omega-3 fatty acids, you can get plenty of them by eating fish once or twice a week. Using the relatively huge amounts of the EFAs found in the supplements over the long term without addressing the underlying cause is just going to create yet another imbalance in your body.

✦ PMS AND THE DIET CONNECTION

What you've read above gives you a pretty good background on how nutrition can affect PMS symptoms and hormone balance. The bottom line is that if you want to cause PMS, eat plenty of high-calorie, high-sugar foods made with refined carbohydrates and hydrogenated or unsaturated vegetable oils. If you want to avoid PMS, avoid those foods. Trans-fatty acids (partially hydrogenated oils) block anti-inflammatory prostaglandins, and sugar stimulates adrenaline, cortisol, and insulin production, all of which will contribute to blocking progesterone and raising cortisol and prolactin levels.

The mainstay of a PMS-free diet is plenty of fresh, organic vegetables and a moderate amount of whole, fresh fruit. We'll get into more details on the optimal hormone balance diet in chapter 14, but right now it's important to stress that just avoiding sugar and refined carbohydrates can have a major impact on PMS symptoms.

Zinc and copper are two important trace minerals whose balance in the body is closely interwoven. An excess or deficiency of either can cause serious health problems. Ellen Grant, M.D., a British hormone researcher and author, believes that the retention of copper and the loss of zinc, which can be caused by estrogen dominance, correlates with the anger and rage experienced by women who have severe PMS. Oral contraceptives are known to lower zinc levels and raise copper levels. As mentioned above, zinc deficiency can also contribute to an imbalance of EFAs that increases inflammation and PMS symptoms. Other symptoms of zinc deficiency include loss of the sense of taste and smell, brittle or peeling fingernails, prematurely graying hair, hair loss, acne, fatigue, infertility, poor memory, blood sugar imbalances, and chronic infections.

Symptoms of excess copper include anxiety, depression, mood swings, diarrhea, nausea and vomiting, achy joints and muscle pain, high cholesterol and blood pressure, and insomnia. Some people believe that anorexia nervosa is associated with excess copper. Severe copper toxicity can cause hallucinations, paranoid schizophrenia, and symptoms of senility.

Deficiencies of magnesium and vitamin B6, both nutrients that are intimately connected with your body's ability to maintain hormone balance, can also contribute to PMS. It's important to take a good multivitamin every day, or if you have a hard time tolerating daily vitamins, at least take them premenstrually. There are many excellent vitamin and mineral formulas specifically made for treating PMS symptoms.

❧ THE EMOTIONAL SIDE OF PMS

One of the reasons that PMS frequently doesn't respond completely to attempts to change it with natural hormones, supplements, diet, and exercise is that there is an emotional component that goes with it that has an underlying and important purpose in a woman's life. Dr. Hanley has worked extensively with this aspect of PMS because she believes that without it full healing often can't take place.

Dr. Hanley approaches PMS, with all its emotional volatility, as an important guide and teacher. She calls it the goddesses' gift. It is a time in a woman's cycle when she is especially sensitive and has access to her deeper levels of intuitive knowing. This knowing is often filled with pain in our culture because of all of the conflict women have with feelings they are not supposed to have. Women are not supposed to have anger. They are not supposed to be anything but sweet and nurturing, and this sets up a pattern of repressed emotions and guilt over those times when anger and frustration do boil over.

The typical woman who visits Dr. Hanley with PMS aggravated or fueled by emotional conflict says, "I'm not myself. I cannot just take it all in stride anymore. I'm angry, I'm agitated, I have really strong feelings, I'm reactive, I'm a witch and a bitch! What is wrong with me?" Dr. Hanley would say, "There's nothing wrong with you!

What you're experiencing is an important teacher, and we'll use all kinds of wonderful tools to help you learn about what's underneath that anger, to appreciate and honor your sensitivity, and to balance your body so that you have control of this phenomenon." PMS helps you to have a moment, or a day, or a week to have access to parts of yourself that are not necessarily sweet and happy or just pretending to be sweet and happy. PMS gives you a window of opportunity for identifying and working with these feelings.

At one time in history menstrual blood was not considered dirty or a "curse"; it was cherished as sacred and used in rituals and to fertilize the fields. A woman who was menstruating went to a special lodge with her sisters where her increased sensitivity and cyclic ability to tap into her deeper knowing was used to help guide the tribe or village. In ancient Greece, menstruating women were consulted as oracles. Their dreams, thoughts, and opinions were highly regarded and seriously considered.

Today a sensitive menstrual woman is regarded as a liability, someone to be feared and avoided. In fact, at any point during the month when a woman expresses anger or irritation, she may be accused of having PMS. If she has a strong opinion she may be accused of being a "ball buster" or of trying to be like a man, as opposed to just being smart or competent. However, sensitive also means more intuitive, more in touch, more creative, more spontaneous, and more unpredictable. When these attributes are expressed and appreciated, first and foremost by the woman herself, they tend to be expressed in a more positive way. When a woman's loved ones also appreciate her more sensitive times, it's a true gift.

PMS may push a woman to understand that she does have limits and that those limits are not shameful; they are to be honored. Women need to recognize for themselves when they are neglected, abused, overworked, unappreciated, and not respected. They need to know that they aren't bad if they can't stay up half the night with a sick child, go to work all day and be competent, and then come home and be cheery, nurturing, and selfless while they cook and do laundry and then stay up half the night again.

Feelings that have been suppressed all month may flare up out of proportion premenstrually. Women who feel free to express and discuss their feelings and to implement their intuitive knowledge have a much better handle on their emotions when they are premenstrual. When women learn to respect and listen to their own intuitive knowledge, they are taking their first step in healing themselves. Dr. Hanley asks women to search for that kernel of truth in their anger, their frustration, their volatility. They can search through dance, journals, painting, sculpture, dream journals, women's groups, the Chinese exercises such as yoga and tai chi, or any other creative form of expression that takes them deeper into themselves. As this process takes place, women learn to be excited and intrigued by their increased sensitivity and to look for the wisdom and creativity available to them.

Women who access valuable knowing through a creative process and their intuition find that if they need to, they can later express this knowing in a more linear, rational, or logical way. Many times, women are parallel processors, processing and integrating a large amount of information at once in a nonlinear, nonlogical way: They just "know." This is a gift and a strength, just as thinking in a linear, logical fashion is a strength (and yes, both men and women have the ability to do both kinds of thinking). The key is to know that when you know, you really do know, even though you may not have an immediate, logical explanation for *why* you know! Men who access their own intuition through their "muse" are tapping into the same way of knowing.

Acknowledging and appreciating the greater sensitivity of a woman's premenstrual time is a core issue that profoundly affects her overall physical, mental, and emotional health and well-being. This is why it's so counterproductive and often destructive to walk into a conventional medical doctor's office with the emotional complaints of PMS. If antidepressants don't fix the problem, you'll be given a "crazy" label, and that results in even more crazy making.

With some personal sleuthing and creativity, and a willingness to keep track of what works and what doesn't, PMS can usually be brought into balance within a few months. If you can find a sympathetic and knowledgeable health care professional to work in partnership with you and help you monitor your progress, that's wonderful. If not, you have all the tools and resources to create healing and balance yourself.

❧ HEALING PMS ❧

What to Do

- Correct estrogen dominance with natural progesterone cream.*
- Take a daily multivitamin/mineral that includes zinc, 10 mg; B complex (all of the B vitamins); vitamin C, 500–1000 mg; magnesium, 300–400 mg; vitamin E, 400 IU daily. In addition, take Vitamin B6, 50 mg daily.
- Eat a plant-based, fiber-rich diet of fresh, organic vegetables and fruits, nuts, seeds, whole grains, and legumes.
- Eat fish at least twice a week.
- Take evening primrose oil or borage oil to treat symptoms (equivalent to 300 mg GLA oils once or twice daily).
- Take an herbal formula for PMS such as the Chinese Bu Tiao or Hsiao Wan or a Western formula that includes some or all of the following herbs: peony root, milk thistle (*Silybum marianum*), *Vitex*, wild yam (*Dioscorea*), dandelion root, yarrow, and nettle.
- Take a liver-supporting and detoxifying herbal formula that includes some or all of the following herbs: *Bupleurum,* milk thistle (*Silybum marianum*), barberry or goldenseal, burdock root, yellow dock, dandelion root.

- Manage stress to avoid chronically high cortisol levels.
- Get some exercise every day.
- Keep a journal and allow yourself to notice the deeper levels of your anger and pain. Seek to resolve unresolved issues the rest of the month.

What to Avoid

- Birth control pills
- Unopposed estrogen
- Situations that cause anovulatory cycles (see Healing the Ovaries box on pages 142–143)
- Sugar and refined carbohydrates
- Rancid unsaturated oils and hydrogenated oils
- Feed-lot meats (eat range-fed, organic meats free of drugs and pesticide residues)
- Pesticides of all kinds
- Chronic stress

*See chapter 16 for details on how to use natural progesterone cream.

Chapter 9

❧

Tired Adrenals Equals a Tired Woman

*U*nderlying many of the symptoms of premenopause syndrome in most women are two tired adrenal glands that have been flogged for years into overproducing the "up" hormones epinephrine, adrenaline, androgens, and cortisols. In Western industrialized societies in general, and in America in particular, we love to be in a high-energy mode, zipping and zooming around and being busy and efficient. What this means in terms of our hormone balance (men and women) is that we exist in a culture that lives off its adrenal function.

The adrenals are two small glands, about the size and shape of a flattened prune, that sit on top of the kidneys. Each adrenal gland is composed of an outer and inner part: the outer cortex and the inner medulla. Both the medulla and the cortex produce important secretions that are part of our stress reactions.

The adrenal medulla plays a role in regulating the sympathetic nervous system: It speeds up the heart rate, narrows blood vessels, and raises blood pressure and blood sugar by secreting two hormones called epinephrine (also called adrenaline) and norepinephrine (noradrenaline). You probably recognize the name epinephrine because synthetic variations of this hormone are found in over-the-counter cold and allergy remedies that work by narrowing blood vessels. Epinephrine (adrenaline) is the hormone secreted when you're under stress. To help you respond to the stress and the release of these hormones, your body simultaneously and quickly speeds up the heart and sends blood flooding into the heart, lungs, muscles, and brain and away from the digestive system; sugar is dumped into the blood in large quantities to provide quick energy; and breathing is faster.

When we're stimulated by epinephrine we tend to be very alert, focused, and energetic. This type of energy is particularly valued in the business world. Some people will work themselves into an anger or fear response just to get a "hit" of epinephrine. The bad news is that epinephrine is not a hormone meant to be used all the time—it's designed to be used in emergencies for short bursts of intense energy. If we're always calling on our epinephrine to get us up and going, eventually we fall prey to an imbalance and our adrenal medulla becomes exhausted.

The adrenal cortex secretes three classes of hormones—glucocorticoids, mineralocorticoids and androgens—which play literally dozens of ongoing roles in regulating bodily functions. While the secretions of the adrenal medulla provide quick and short-term responses to immediate stress, the adrenal cortex hormones provide longer-term responses for stress and homeostasis, which is the maintenance of balance in bodily functions. The adrenal cortex hormones are often considered essential for life. Animals with their adrenal glands removed will survive for a long time if maintained in an environment providing proper nutrition and freedom from stress. However, if put to any significant stress such as infection, trauma, hunger, or fatigue, they will quickly die. Adrenal cortical hormones are essential for life because life, as we know it, is stressful.

An important class of glucocorticoids are the cortisols, which play a role in regulating blood sugar; the movement of carbohydrates, proteins, and fats in and out of cells; inflammation; and muscle function. Chronic stress causes chronically elevated levels of cortisol. The symptoms of too much cortisol include:

- Weight gain (especially around the midsection)
- Blood sugar imbalances (a good clue to these symptoms is whether you're a sugar junkie and/or get shaky when you don't eat regularly)
- Thinning or papery skin
- Muscle wasting
- Memory loss

Recent research has shown that people who have high cortisol levels year after year from leading overly stressful lives age faster and have more deterioration in the part of the brain called the hippocampus, which is responsible for memory and spatial navigation.

It's also interesting to note that excess estrogen causes a decrease in cortisol levels in rats. In this case, more of the releasing hormone that tells the adrenals to make more cortisol is secreted by the hypothalamus in the brain, but the adrenals don't respond as readily. This could indicate yet another connection between estrogen dominance and the symptoms of premenopause, created by cortisol deficiency.

It's possible for a woman to have both the symptoms of excess cortisol, from years of chronic stress, and the symptoms of adrenal exhaustion, which is the inability to maintain adequate production of adrenal steroids. The symptoms of cortisol deficiency are included in the symptoms of tired adrenals listed below.

The mineralocorticoids, especially aldosterone, regulate the balance of minerals in the cells, mainly sodium and potassium, but magnesium is also affected. Stress triggers the release of aldosterone, which raises blood pressure by its action on body cells to hold on to sodium and lose potassium and magnesium. Long-term release of stress-level mineralocorticoids can cause a potassium deficiency and a magnesium imbalance, as well as chronic water retention and high blood pressure. Magnesium loss is an exceedingly important risk factor in maintaining our overall health.

The adrenal cortex also makes all of the sex hormones, but in very small amounts. One cortical hormone, DHEA, which is weakly androgenic, is made in large amounts in both men and women; its production is greater than that of any of the other corticosteroids. Both cortisol and DHEA, and how to take them as supplements, are discussed in more detail in chapter 17.

Over many years of constantly having to push to keep up with demands of chronic stress, the delicate feedback system that controls the secretion of adrenal hormones can go out of balance. If the adrenals swell, as they often do when overworked for years, the inflammation causes adrenal cells to die off. These glands have enormous reserves of energy, and until 90 percent of the mass of the glands has died, outright symptoms may not appear.

If you have some or all of the following symptoms, you may be suffering from what is known in the medical world as mild adrenal insufficiency—what we like to call tired adrenals.

- Constant fatigue, especially in the mornings when trying to get out of bed and after exercise
- Muscle weakness
- Low blood pressure
- Low metabolism coupled with decreased thyroid function
- Excess pigmentation, which may look like tanning or dark freckles on the skin
- Allergies and/or asthma

- Low reserves for coping with stress—if anything doesn't happen on schedule, you're unable to meet demands and have to take time to recuperate
- Irregular menstrual cycles, fibrocystic breasts, anovulatory periods, infertility
- Difficulty resisting infectious illnesses like flu and upper respiratory infection
- Depression caused by the constant fatigue, weakness, and inability to cope with stress

The balance of the sex hormones is inextricably bound up with the balance of the adrenal hormones. As you read in chapter 2, cholesterol is a precursor to all of the adrenal cortex and sex hormones, and progesterone is a precursor to aldosterone, the mineralocorticoid that regulates fluids in your cells, and cortisol. This means that aldosterone and cortisol are made from progesterone. Now that you know how important aldosterone and cortisol are to bodily functions, you can imagine what havoc a deficiency of progesterone can wreak on hormone balance and bodily functions. A drop in progesterone can cause a concurrent drop in cortisol production, creating a vicious cycle.

The adrenal cortex is also capable of making progesterone, principally for its precursor role in making corticosteroids, but many women are so stressed out trying to work, raise children, and be wives all at the same time that by the time they're premenopausal their adrenal glands are just plain tired and they are unable to make progesterone anywhere in the body.

The thyroid gland and the adrenals work very closely together. If a woman's adrenals are weak, her thyroid might slow down to compensate, and vice versa. This scenario is what often causes low blood pressure, a much more common problem in women than in men. The best way to find out if you have low blood pressure caused by adrenal dysfunction is to have your blood pressure taken when you are lying down and then after standing up. If your blood pressure is normal, the change from lying down to standing up will cause an initial drop and then a quick rise in blood pressure. If your blood pressure is low, the response is considerably slower, and you might feel dizzy, unsteady, or have blurry vision when you stand. However, even if you don't have this response, your blood pressure still may be low.

Conventional medical doctors seem to have forgotten that low blood pressure is not normal. High blood pressure has gotten such a bad name, thanks to years of massive advertising campaigns for drugs to lower it, that we tend to forget that low blood pressure can also cause problems and is a symptom of dysfunction in the body, usually poorly functioning adrenal glands. We wonder how many women visit their doctor, get a low blood pressure reading, which is ignored, and then get put on an antidepressant because they complain that they are tired and depressed.

A "normal" blood pressure reading for an adult is 130 (systolic) over 85 (diastolic), also shown as 130/85 mm Hg (millimeters of mercury, under pressure). Blood pressure rises as we age, so people over the age of 60 may have "normal" blood pressure as high as 180/100.

One of the best cures for low blood pressure caused by tired adrenals is salt. It's a misconception that salt is bad for everyone—excessive salt can create high blood pressure in *some* people. Using a moderate amount of salt is perfectly healthy, and it's unhealthy to eliminate it from the diet. Dr. Hanley asks her patients to use sea salt, because it contains a naturally occurring mixture of salt and minerals.

Women with tired adrenals usually get a lot of benefit from using natural progesterone cream. They may also need to use some natural cortisol in small doses to regain hormone balance. This is discussed in detail in chapter 17. Licorice is a very adrenal-supportive herb but needs to be used in moderation because it can also raise estrogen levels. You can use licorice in tea, tincture, or capsule form, following the directions on the container.

The single best remedy for restoring tired adrenals is rest. If you have tired adrenals and you try to prop them up with supplemental hormones and herbs without resting, you may get away with it for a while, but eventually that will stop working too and you'll create disease in your body. You need to do both if you want to heal. Rest means relief from stress, plenty of sleep, and plenty of play. And that means gentle play—no bungee jumping! Activities such as gardening, playing the guitar, or walking your dog are all examples of exercise that are both active and restful.

❖ HEALING THE ADRENALS ❖

What to Do

- Use natural progesterone cream to support adrenal hormone production.*
- Manage chronic stress more effectively through creative outlets, exercise, counseling, journal writing, and so on.
- Get enough sleep and play time.
- Take an adrenal-supporting herbal formula that includes some or all of the following herbs: licorice root, *Bupleurum,* peony root, wild yam (*Dioscorea*), Siberian ginseng, smilax (sarsaparilla).
- Increase salt if you have low blood pressure (use sea salt).
- Check your thyroid symptoms and levels.
- Take a good multivitamin/mineral supplement daily that includes the B complex vitamins (all of the B vitamins); magnesium, 300–400 mg daily; vitamin C, 500–1,000 mg daily; vitamin E, 400 IU daily; an extra 50 mg of vitamin B6.
- Check your hormone levels and supplement with DHEA if needed, 5–10 mg daily or every other day.
- Have your doctor check your cortisol levels and supplement natural hydrocortisone in small,

physiologic doses if needed, 5–10 mg, 1 to 3 times daily, with meals.

What to Avoid

- Chronic stress
- Stimulating herbs such as ephedra, and caffeine
- Sugar and refined carbohydrates
- Dairy products
- Feed-lot meats (eat only range-fed, organic meats that are free of drugs and pesticide residues)

*See chapter 16 for details on how to use natural progesterone cream.

Chapter 10

❖

Other Premenopause Syndrome Symptoms and Solutions

*I*t's difficult to describe the relief that women feel when they balance their hormones and come out of the ill effects of premenopause syndrome. One of the best descriptions we've read comes from a woman named Linda, who has turned a longer version of the following letter into a brochure and is handing it out to any woman who will take it:

> Mood swings, chronic fatigue, foggy thinking, depression, leg cramps, migraine headaches, heavy painful periods, anemia, endometriosis, shooting back and extremity pain, water retention and bloating, sleep dysfunction, anxiety attacks, thinning hair, allergies, chronic sinus infections, fever

blisters, acne, dry skin, infertility, hypoglycemic symptoms, and fibroids are only a few of the many symptoms that dominated my life for years.

Those years were so challenging physically and emotionally, I thought I'd never survive! At the age of 30, doctors were giving me every conflicting diagnosis in the world, taking my money for doing so, and yet leaving me without any help or suggestions for getting help. I saw gynecologists, endocrinologists, dermatologists, neurologists, and assorted other "-ologists." Their comments ranged from "The tests show that you are perfectly healthy. It must be in your head, take this Xanax," to "Something is definitely wrong, but I don't know what it is." Emotionally I felt like I was on the verge of a mental breakdown. I felt very alone.

Finally I drove four hours to see a specialist who put me on synthetic estrogen, a progestin, and testosterone. At first, I felt so good I thought this was the miracle for which I had been praying. But within two years of starting this treatment the symptoms came back. The doctor's answer was to continue increasing my dosage until I was at the maximum level: six implants, the patch, and shots in between. I went from seeing him every six months to every three months. The hormones were only effective for two months, and the last month before I could get back for more implants I felt emotionally and physically as if I had been thrown off a ten-story building. I lived my life surviving from office visit to office visit. I was having constant back pain, heavy bleeding, anemia, and varying degrees of all my old symptoms, some worse than before. My pap smears began indicating precancerous cells. This went on for about a year before I finally agreed to have a hysterectomy. The surgery alleviated the bleeding, anemia, and back pain for obvious reasons—my uterus was three times its normal size and density! However, all the other symptoms continued.

It was three years after my surgery before I learned about natural progesterone and began using it. After a brief period of withdrawal from synthetic hormones, the only hormone I have used during the past four years is a natural progesterone cream. I also have combined this with a balanced diet, exercise, and nutritional supplements. My life has changed dramatically. Today, I feel like I did when I was in my 20s: I have energy; can think clearly; no depression; my skin is wonderful; I am losing weight; can sleep at night; no more migraines; my hair has stopped falling out; the dark facial hair is disappearing; and my allergies have disappeared. No more antihistamines! This is the answer to my prayers. My family is glad to have the "real me" back.

It's sad that Linda's story is not all that unusual. It is very common to hear stories from women whose symptoms are less severe but who are suffering from similar problems. Dr. Lee has been (wrongly) accused of talking only about natural progesterone cream as if it were the magic solution to a woman's every problem, but this letter demonstrates why. Progesterone cream is certainly not a magic potion. But it is the best remedy we've found so far to counteract the effects of living in a state of xeno-hormone excess. We do not naturally need to supplement progesterone. Mother Nature has equipped us to live a long, healthy robust life given a wholesome environment. If we were living in a stress-free, unpolluted world, if we were eating whole, fresh organic foods, and if we got plenty of outdoor exercise, we probably wouldn't ever need progesterone.

✤ ACT EARLY TO PREVENT SYMPTOMS LATER

A woman's hormone balance can begin to shift anywhere from her late twenties to her late forties, depending on a variety of factors. Symptoms do increase with age and as you get closer to menopause, especially if you ignore them early on. Twenty percent of women don't have any premenopausal or menopausal symptoms at all. Our guess is that if you only polled women who still had a uterus and ovaries, the number would be higher.

Individual factors that can affect your hormone balance include heredity, at what age you began menstruating, whether you have been pregnant, and how many children you have given birth to, if any. The quality of your environment, from the time of your conception to the present, is important. Environment includes such broad considerations as exposure to air pollution and pesticides, whether your diet emphasizes whole food or junk food, stress levels, physical abuse, sexual abuse, and drug and alcohol abuse. Even low self-esteem, which creates an environment of chronic inner stress, can affect your hormone levels.

The earlier in your life that you detect symptoms of premenopause syndrome and act to balance them, the easier it will be to stay in balance as you approach menopause. Even if menopause is a decade or more away, how you treat yourself now will play a pivotal role in how you feel later. If your hormones and your life have been out of balance for decades, in the five or ten years before menopause the symptoms of imbalance will become extreme, because you no longer have the reserves of youth to draw on.

This concept of prevention is a tough sell to a woman in her mid-thirties who is roaring through her life with the pedal to the metal, busy taking care of everyone else. If you need some inspiration to take care of yourself, ask women in their fifties and sixties what they would have done differently, and you'll find they are nearly unanimous in their wish that they had paid more attention to their own needs.

If you are interested in delving more deeply into the specific emotional and psychological patterns that can precipitate health problems in a woman's body, the books of Christiane Northrup and Caroline Myss are recommended. (See the Recommended Reading section in the back of the book.)

❧ TURNING DOWN THE THERMOSTAT

Biochemist David Zava likes to compare what happens to a woman's hormone levels as she ages to turning down a thermostat: All involved systems, from the brain to the uterus, are down-regulating. If you maintain balance in your life, it will be a gradual, barely noticeable process. If you're out of balance, all of the systems will not be getting the message that down-regulation is in process, and they will, in effect, be shouting at each other to try to provoke a response, causing night sweats and hot flashes. Your brain will secrete large amounts of regulatory hormones in an attempt to get the ovaries to release higher levels of hormones. Your ovaries may be asleep for a few months, deaf to the shouts of the brain, and then wake up and respond to the shouting from the brain with a great surge of hormones. It is this type of biochemical overreaction or underreaction that causes high libido, low libido, acne, allergies, tender breasts, water retention, insomnia, and mood swings (to name a few) and makes you wonder if you have reentered adolescence.

When a premenopausal woman enters a doctor's office with these complaints, she is highly likely to leave with a prescription for estrogen or a birth control pill, which is probably the last thing in the world she needs. The doctor may check her estradiol levels and her FSH and LH levels but will rarely check her progesterone levels. Her estrogen level may come out lower than "normal," but to supplement it is going to cause a world of troubles and doesn't allow the body to proceed in its natural premenopausal process of down-regulation. And to supplement estrogen without progesterone, which is once again becoming an increasingly common practice, is to write a prescription for cancer. Chances are excellent that a premenopausal woman prescribed unopposed estrogen will have an abnormal pap test within a year, and her risk of breast cancer is considerably increased. If she has an abnormal pap smear, her doctor will immediately suggest removing her uterus. Please don't go there! (See chapters 6 and 7.)

PMS is one of the most common, disturbing, and complex symptoms of premenopause syndrome, but chapter 8 has laid the groundwork for you to put together your own PMS cure. In this chapter we'll give you more pieces of the premenopause puzzle by describing other common premenopause syndrome symptoms and what might be causing them. How you put the pieces together for yourself will be unique to you.

❖ PAINFUL, SWOLLEN BREASTS AND BREAST CYSTS

Painful, swollen, and lumpy breasts are a common PMS symptom but can be present without PMS. Estimates are that 70 percent of women suffer from this problem at one time or another, and it's one of the most common reasons a woman makes a doctor's appointment. As time goes on, this symptom may develop into what is known as fibrocystic breasts, or the formation of tender lumps called cysts that last throughout the month. Cysts are benign, or noncancerous, but they are painful, and their presence makes it almost impossible to detect a cancerous lump. Cancerous lumps are almost never painful.

Using natural progesterone cream virtually always resolves the problem, and it can be rubbed directly on the breasts for faster relief. (See chapter 16 for details on how to use natural progesterone.) Progesterone works so well because estrogen dominance and the progestins found in birth control pills stimulate the growth of breast tissue and the retention of fluids, both of which contribute to the swelling.

At one time it was thought that fibrocystic breasts predisposed women to cancer, but that turned out to be inaccurate. However, premenstrually painful and lumpy breasts indicate chronic estrogen dominance, and that is a risk factor for breast cancer because it means the breasts are exposed to unopposed estrogen on a regular basis. Breast cancer is covered in detail in chapter 12.

The dietary advice given in the chapter on PMS applies here too. Be sure you're taking a good multivitamin supplement premenstrually that includes 400 IU vitamin E, 300 to 400 mg magnesium, and 50 mg vitamin B6. Some women find that coffee drinking aggravates painful breasts so it's worth giving it up to find out whether that's a culprit. Either way, giving up coffee is good for your overall health and well-being.

If you have cysts, once they have cleared up, you can reduce the progesterone dose to find the smallest dose that is still effective each month, and continue the treatment as needed through menopause. This treatment is simple, safe, inexpensive, successful, and natural.

❖ HEALING PAINFUL BREASTS ❖

What to Do

- Use some natural progesterone cream to balance estrogen dominance.*
- Take a good multivitamin/mineral daily that includes zinc, 10 mg; the B complex vitamins (all of the B vitamins); vitamin E, 400 IU; magnesium, 300–400 mg; vitamin C, 500–1,000 mg.
- Use a liver-supporting and detoxifying herbal formula that includes some or all of the following herbs: *Bupleurum,* milk thistle (*Silybum marianum*), barberry or goldenseal, burdock root, yellow dock, dandelion root.
- Use a woman's herbal formula that includes some or all of the following herbs: *Vitex,* blue cohosh, wild yam (*Dioscorea*), dong quai.

What to Avoid

- Estrogen dominance and unopposed estrogen
- Caffeine in general and coffee in particular
- Dairy products

- Feed-lot meats (eat only range-fed organic meats free of drugs and pesticide residues)

*See chapter 16 for details on how to use natural progesterone cream.

✦ IRREGULAR AND HEAVY MENSTRUAL CYCLES

"My periods are sometimes very light, sometimes very heavy, and sometimes come early or late. What should I do?" This is one of the most common questions a premenopausal woman has. Your doctor defines irregular periods as amennorhea (no period), dysmenorrhea (painful periods), menorrhagia (lasting too long), hypermenorrhea (heavy bleeding), metrorrhagia (bleeding between periods), and polymenorrhea (having periods too often).

Up to the age of forty, some 90 percent of women have regular periods. Between the age of forty and fifty only 10 percent of women have regular cycles. Only 10 percent of women experience an abrupt end to menstruation. In most it is preceded by irregular periods. In other words, it is quite normal to have irregular periods when you are premenopausal!

It is also common for a physician to assume that there is something wrong with a woman who doesn't fit into the so-called normal menstrual cycle of 28 to 30 days.

Chronobiologist William Hrushesky, who has closely studied the timing of women's hormone cycles, has found that it is perfectly normal for a woman's cycle to be as short as 18 days or as long as 36 days. According to Hrushesky, the number of days from the day your period begins to the day you ovulate can vary considerably. Women may ovulate anywhere from days 3 to 14 of their cycle. Once ovulation has taken place, the number of days until menstruation tends to be a consistent 14 days.

The vast majority of the time, irregularly timed periods are yet another sign that you are deficient in progesterone, the result of not ovulating every month, because your body isn't getting the proper hormonal signals to begin the last phase of the menstrual cycle. Remember, shedding of the blood-rich endometrial (uterine) lining is triggered primarily by the fall of progesterone levels 12 to 15 days or so after ovulation. If you are not ovulating, you are not making any significant amount of progesterone, and therefore there will be no fall of progesterone to trigger a proper shedding or sloughing. When it does shed, it may not do it completely, or flow may be heavy one day and light the next.

Irregularly timed periods are sometimes caused by ovarian cysts (see chapter 7). Some studies indicate that having your tubes tied (tubal ligation) increases menstrual irregularities.

There are illnesses that can cause irregularly timed periods, including hyperthyroidism or hypothyroidism (high or low thyroid), Cushing's disease (overactive adrenal glands), and a dysfunctional pituitary gland. Some prescription drugs can cause irregular periods, including cortisols (prednisone), digoxin, anticoagulants (warfarin), anticholinergic drugs, and drugs that affect the brain such as the benzodiazepines (Valium, Ativan) and the selective serotonin reuptake inhibitors (SSRIs) such as Prozac and Effexor.

When Dr. Hanley sees a younger woman with irregular bleeding, she will often begin treatment by changing her diet (increasing fiber and vegetables, decreasing dairy products and junk food), adding a multivitamin, and also adding 100 mg vitamin B6 and 200 mg magnesium twice daily for the last two weeks of the cycle, to support progesterone production and decrease estrogen.

The standard medical treatment for irregular bleeding is to prescribe the synthetic progestin Provera (medroxy-progesterone) or a birth control pill. You don't need to suffer the miseries of Provera and birth control pills; you can simply use some natural progesterone cream. It's important after the first month or two to use the smallest possible dose of progesterone that will relieve your symptoms to allow your body to continue its normal down-regulation of hormones.

In women who prefer to be treated with herbs first, Dr. Hanley finds that the herb *Vitex* (chaste tree) often works well to normalize cycles. Research indicates that *Vitex* stimulates the hypothalamus gland in the brain to increase the production of luteinizing hormone (LH), which is secreted by the brain to stimulate the production of progesterone (possibly stimulating the release of the egg from the follicle). Dr. Hanley has found that women with low LH tend to have a hard time getting pregnant and tend to have bleeding and cycling problems and PMS.

If you are bleeding on and off through the month and you're not sure when your period is beginning and ending, use your intuition and pick a day that you will call day 1 of your menstrual cycle. Begin taking the progesterone on day 12, and depending on the length of your normal menstrual cycle, stop taking it between days 21 and 28, and start again on day 12. After a couple of months of doing this, your periods should become much more regular. If you have a fibroid, it may take up to six months before your periods are regular again.

Bleeding or spotting throughout the menstrual cycle is most often caused by the use of birth control pills, an IUD, progestins, or sometimes by a fibroid or an ovarian cyst. If it's an ovarian cyst, the bleeding is often accompanied by pelvic pain and will usually resolve itself in a month or two. Using progesterone for two weeks in the middle of your cycle may help resolve the cyst more quickly.

It is normal to skip a period now and then in the few years just before menopause. An absence of periods can also be caused by heavy exercise, stress, a fast gain or loss of weight, excessive androgens (male hormones), and ovarian cysts. Some of the oral contraceptives are so androgenic that they can cause missed periods and facial hair.

Heavy Bleeding: For some women heavy monthly bleeding comes with the premenopausal territory, regardless of progesterone use. It is a frequent complaint in the year or two just before menopause and is a very common reason cited by doctors for recommending a hysterectomy.

Heavy bleeding can be directly caused by a fibroid or an enlarged uterus (see chapter 6), but it is usually caused simply by too much estrogen stimulating the uterus to keep growing and growing.

Weight gain correlates somewhat with heavy bleeding, which makes sense since we know that the fat cells are producing estrogen, along with whatever is produced by the ovaries. The more estrogen that is present, the more the uterine lining will be stimulated to grow the blood-rich lining, and the heavier the bleeding will be.

Dr. Hanley has had great success treating heavy bleeding by using very high doses of progesterone cream, 100 to 200 mg daily, for a few weeks, and then gradually reducing the dosage. The best way to minimize heavy bleeding in general, however, is to allow your hormone levels to drop the way nature intended them to. You can use a little bit of progesterone to balance estrogen dominance symptoms, but don't use any estrogen unless you have clear estrogen deficiency symptoms such as hot flashes, night sweats, and vaginal dryness. (It is unlikely that you would have heavy bleeding if you have estrogen-deficiency symptoms.) Also avoid foods that are likely to be tainted with estrogens such as dairy products and red meat, and eat organic fruits and vegetables as much as possible to avoid the xenoestrogens found in pesticides.

In a small study of heavy bleeding, the NSAID (non-steroidal anti-inflammatory drug) naproxen, a close relative of ibuprofen, was given (500 mg twice daily) during the first three days of the menstrual cycle. Women taking the naproxen reported their bleeding was reduced by about one third. Since the ibuprofen-type drugs are very hard on the stomach (taking them just two or three days a month can cause chronic stomach pain), you're probably better off using evening primrose oil or borage oil (follow dosage instructions on the container), which contain the essential fatty acids (EFAs) that block the same prostaglandins as the NSAIDs, only more selectively and without the side effects.

❧ HEALING IRREGULAR BLEEDING ❧

What to Do

- Balance estrogen dominance or excess estrogen by using a small dose of natural progesterone cream.*
- Eat a plant-based, fiber-rich diet (at least 20–30 g fiber daily).
- Take vitamin B6, 50–100 mg daily for up to two weeks per month.
- Take magnesium, 200–400 mg daily.
- Use evening primrose oil or borage oil to treat symptoms.
- For weak, irregular to absent menses, take an herbal formula that includes some or all of the following herbs: false unicorn root, ginger,

licorice root, dong quai, *Vitex*, wild yam (*Dioscorea*), burdock root, smilax (*sarsaparilla*), Siberian ginseng, rue.

- For spotting outside of menses or early menses, take an herbal formula that includes some or all of the following herbs: *Vitex*, blue cohosh, licorice root, false unicorn root, burdock root, motherwort (*Leonuris cardiaca*), cinnamon, red raspberry, ginger.

What to Avoid

- Dairy products
- Junk food, including caffeine, sugar and refined carbohydrates
- Feed-lot meats (eat only range-fed organic meats free of drugs and pesticide residues)

*See chapter 16 for details on how to use natural progesterone cream.

❖ INFERTILITY

There is an epidemic of infertility among women in their thirties that we believe is largely caused by the high levels of xenohormones in the environment, which affect the reproductive tracts of both women and men from conception on. Exposure to xenohormones in the womb can cause a lifetime of reproductive problems. Oral contraceptives, contraceptive implants and shots, and intrauterine devices (IUDs) also contribute to infertility.

For example, daughters of women who were given the synthetic estrogen DES (diethylstilbestrol) during pregnancy have an increased risk of vaginal and cervical cancer, miscarriage, ectopic pregnancy, stillbirth, premature labor, and sterility. DES sons have a higher risk of genital birth defects, sterility, infertility, and testicular cancer. DES is no longer given to pregnant women (though it is given to livestock that we eat, including cows and pigs, to fatten them up for market), but it is a tragic example of the potency of hormonal influences on the developing fetus. As Dr. Ellen Grant points out in her book *The Bitter Pill: How Safe Is the Perfect Contraceptive?*, if vaginal cancers in young women hadn't been extremely rare to begin with, the connection between DES and reproductive abnormalities might never have been made. It's probable that the high risk of breast cancer for women and the increasing risk of testicular cancer for men is caused by exposure to xenohormones, which have become so prevalent in the environment that it's impossible to determine that they are the cause. Because no one lives in a xenohormone-free environment, there's simply no basis for comparison.

Solid connections *have* been made between xenohormones and infertility in birds, fish, reptiles, and mammals. The doses necessary to cause reproductive abnormalities in an egg and infertility in an adult are extremely small.

Dr. Hanley believes that high levels of xenohormones

in the environment are reducing the ability of the brain to send out the hormone-stimulating substances that cause the manufacture of hormones, as well as the ability of the ovaries and the testicles to respond. In effect, the high levels of background xenohormones we're exposed to daily send a message to the hypothalamus that it doesn't need to send out signals to the ovary to begin the ovulation process. The drugs used most frequently by fertility clinics mimic the effect of the signals from the hypothalamus to the ovary.

Anovulatory cycles, in which ovulation does not occur, are very common in women even starting in their early twenties, which is a new phenomenon. Even as recently as ten to fifteen years ago, it was not normal to see frequent anovulatory cycles until a woman was in her forties. Anovulatory menstrual cycles can be verified by checking serum or saliva progesterone levels the week following supposed ovulation. A low reading indicates lack of ovulation and the need to supplement with natural progesterone. (Remember, even if you don't ovulate, you will most often still menstruate.)

Women with a history of miscarriage should begin using progesterone cream as soon as they know they have ovulated, to supplement their own progesterone and offset any environmental estrogen effects. (Using progesterone before ovulation can create a hormonal signal that tells the brain not to ovulate.)

There are many types of ovulation testing kits on the market. One easy way to tell is that your temperature will go up approximately one degree Fahrenheit when you ovulate, which you can tell by taking your temperature under your armpit before you get out of bed in the morning.

If you want to be pregnant and you're using progesterone cream, it's very important to keep using progesterone until you find out whether you're pregnant. (You can take a pregnancy test a few days after your period would normally be due.) The sudden drop in progesterone levels created if you stop using the cream can cause what is, in effect, an abortion, by bringing on menstruation. This is the same concept used in the so-called morning-after pill, only in that case a very potent synthetic progestin is used in high doses.

If you find out that you're not pregnant, stop taking the progesterone on day 28 of your cycle or whenever the last day of your cycle normally occurs. If you *are* pregnant, keep using the progesterone every day in normal doses. It's fine to use it throughout your pregnancy, and it's important not to stop it suddenly until your third trimester when the placenta is making so much that it won't notice if there's a drop of 15 to 30 mg a day. Research by British hormone researcher Katherina Dalton, M.D., indicates that babies born to mothers who used natural progesterone during pregnancy are normal—and, in fact, are larger, calmer, and smarter.

Infertility clinics are booming because so many women are delaying having children and fertility declines steadily with age. Only 11 percent of women age thirty-five or older were childless in 1975. In 1991, 21 percent of women in that age group were childless. The pursuit of fertility through a fertility clinic can be an expensive, complicated process with months and months of erratic side effects from fertility drugs. We now know that fertility drugs that stimulate ovarian function, such as Clomid, significantly increase your risk of ovarian cancer. If you must use them, please don't use them for more than one or two cycles. It's very difficult for a doctor to tell a woman who desperately wants a child that if she uses fertility drugs she has a higher risk of contracting this very deadly cancer, but that is the truth of it, and it needs to be known.

Why are estrogen dominance and infertility related? The answer is that often progesterone deficiency leads to elevated FSH levels, which lead to increased estrogen production. If the follicles are unable to release an egg, no pregnancy results. If the follicle produces an egg and fertilization takes place but the follicle (now the corpus luteum) is unable to sustain continued progesterone production, the conceptus cannot survive.

Before you begin the expensive and often unsuccessful process of working with a fertility clinic, we recommend that you read Dr. Lee's first book, *What Your Doctor May Not Tell You about Menopause,* which will give you a detailed look at how your hormones work.

Dr. Lee had a number of patients in his practice who had been unable to conceive. For two to four months he had them use natural progesterone from days 5 to 26 in the cycle (stopping on day 26 to bring on menstruation). Using the progesterone prior to ovulation effectively suppressed ovulation. After a few months of this, he had them stop progesterone use. If you still have follicles left, they seem to respond to a few months of suppression with enthusiasm—the successful maturation and release of an egg. His patients, some of whom had been trying to conceive for years, had very good luck conceiving with this method. He even has a few children named after him!

Using progesterone prior to ovulation can suppress ovulation. In a normal menstrual cycle, the release of progesterone by one ovary functions as a signal to the other ovary not to ovulate—nature's brilliant plan for avoiding multiple births. If you're using progesterone cream prior to ovulation, chances are good both ovaries will interpret its presence as a sign that the other ovary has ovulated, thus effectively suppressing ovulation.

When Dr. Hanley sees a woman who is having trouble getting pregnant and who also has low levels of LH, she will often prescribe the herb *Vitex* (follow directions on the container), which apparently stimulates the hypothalamus gland in the brain to produce LH. This gentle herbal push is often enough to inspire the ovaries to release an egg.

❧ HEALING INFERTILITY ❧

What to Do

- Stimulate ovulation (see Healing the Ovaries box on pages 142–143).
- If estrogen-dominance symptoms are present, use some natural progesterone cream to restore balance.*

- Use the herb *Vitex* every day, including during menses, for at least three months (unless you become pregnant; then stop).

What to Avoid

- Birth control pills (they can cause infertility)
- Unopposed estrogen
- Talcum powder in the genital region
- Pesticides of all kinds
- Junk foods including caffeine, sugar, and refined carbohydrates

*See chapter 16 for details on how to use natural progesterone cream.

❖ HEADACHES

Estrogen causes swelling in the brain the same way it does in the breasts. Enlarged blood vessels in the brain cause most migraine headaches. Estrogen can also deplete magnesium levels, which makes arteries more susceptible to spasm, a common cause of other types of headaches. For many women, it's that simple. If you have premenstrual headaches, progesterone cream and magnesium will usually cure them within three menstrual cycles.

Although regular coffee drinking is not recommended, a cup or two of full-strength coffee along with an ice pack on the sides of the forehead can very effectively ward off a migraine headache. Both the caffeine and the ice cause blood vessels to constrict.

❧ HEALING HEADACHES ❧

What to Do

- If estrogen-dominance symptoms are present, and/or headaches occur premenstrually, use some natural progesterone cream to restore balance.*
- Take magnesium, 300–400 mg before bed. You can try taking up to 800 mg daily, 400 mg in the morning and 400 mg before bed. If it gives you diarrhea, take less.
- Try an elimination diet to see if an allergic reaction to food is causing the headaches. Some of the most common headache-causing foods include chocolate, nuts, caffeine, dairy products, soy, and wheat. (See chapter 14 for details on the elimination diet.)

*See chapter 16 for details on how to use natural progesterone cream.

❖ YEAST INFECTIONS

There are few women who have never had a yeast infection, which is an overgrowth of a bacteria called *Candida albicans* that is found in the mouth, the intestines, and the vagina. A *Candida* overgrowth causes vaginal itching, redness, white cottage-cheese-like vaginal discharge, and may cause painful intercourse. Normal beneficial bacteria in the gut and vagina (also called probiotics) inhibit *Candida*. A *Candida* overgrowth is primarily caused by taking antibiotics that kill both beneficial and harmful bacteria and by pH imbalances in the vagina. The pH imbalances can be caused by douching, too much sugar in the diet, and frequent intercourse (the ejaculate reduces the acidity of the vagina, creating a friendlier environment for sperm—and for *Candida*). Estrogen dominance can also be a cause of *Candida*, because it increases the amount of glucose (sugar) found in vaginal mucus, which facilitates *Candida* growth. On the other hand, normal estrogen levels are protective against *Candida*. Estriol is particularly effective in restoring normal protective mucus, normal pH, and clearing of harmful pathogens in the vagina. Normal levels of progesterone also play a role in inhibiting yeast, probably by increasing secretory IgA (immune globulin), whereas abnormally high levels promote yeast growth.

The quickest and easiest way to treat a yeast infection if you catch it early is with a twice-daily douche of 1 to 2 cups of apple cider vinegar diluted in 1 quart of water. This raises the acidity of the vagina, creating a hostile environment for the *Candida*. Some women also insert a probiotic gelatin capsule into their vaginas. Probiotics are "friendly" bacteria, such as acidophilus, which keep *Candida* in check. The gelatin capsule dissolves and provides beneficial bacteria that will counter the *Candida*. Probiotics also come in liquid form, which can be used in a douche by mixing ¼ cup probiotics with 1 quart water. (See chapter 14 for more on probiotics.) You can find probiotic supplements at your local health food store in the refrigerated section.

There are also numerous products available both at your health food store and your drugstore that change vaginal pH. It's not necessary to use the antifungal yeast medications unless the infection is very advanced and other methods haven't worked. However, if the yeast infection hasn't cleared up in a week or so with the above treatments, it's a good idea to work with a health care professional to find out what else might be underlying the infection.

❖ HEALING YEAST INFECTIONS ❖

What to Do

- Maintain hormone balance: Excess estrogen or deficient progesterone can contribute to a yeast infection.
- Douche with 1 to 2 cups of apple cider vinegar diluted in 1 quart of water to restore pH, and/or

a probiotic douche or capsule to restore beneficial bacteria.
- If you're having frequent intercourse, douche with the above every few days to avoid a yeast infection.

What to Avoid

- Commercial douches
- Sugar and refined carbohydrates
- Birth control pills
- Antibiotics

❧ AUTOIMMUNE DISEASES

Women are afflicted with autoimmune diseases at a much higher rate than men, which is a good clue that female hormone balance is involved in some way. The onset of autoimmune disorders occurs most often in middle-aged women—the time of life when estrogen dominance becomes common. Hashimoto's thyroiditis, Sjögren's disease, Graves' disease, and lupus all are not only more common in women but also appear to be related to estrogen supplementation or estrogen dominance. Recent studies have shown that women who use HRT containing estrogen are more likely to get lupus. Birth control pills also cause autoimmune diseases by causing the body to form antibodies to its own hormones.

Progesterone can often help ease the symptoms of autoimmune diseases, but it's best to work with an experienced health care professional, such as a naturopath, who can address the whole body. Some clinicians have reported excellent results using DHEA to treat lupus, but there are no studies yet to confirm these reports.

❖ WEIGHT GAIN

Weight gain is a huge issue for premenopausal women. We live in a culture that worships a thin, boy-like body with long legs and large breasts, but the vast majority of women don't look anything like this. We also live in a culture that teaches women to get what they want in the world with their bodies and their sexuality. No wonder we have women starving themselves and taking dangerous drugs to lose weight, and no wonder many women become depressed when they begin to gain weight in their thirties or forties.

Sharon was typical of many women her age. After having her second child in her late thirties she gained twenty-five pounds and just couldn't seem to lose it, no matter what she did. When she went back to work she had to buy a whole new wardrobe. Although she was juggling a full-time job, two children, a marriage, a dog, a cat, and a demanding new home, Sharon began to squeeze in at least three or four sessions a week at the gym to try to get her weight down. For the first few weeks she felt great, but then she began almost collapsing with heavy fatigue after she exercised. She found herself bingeing on ice cream and fatty foods and gaining more weight than ever. When she went to her physician for help, he told her she was depressed and gave her an antidepressant, which seemed to help for a couple of weeks but made her feel edgy and angry.

Sharon is typical of the woman who desperately fights her weight gain, burns herself out in the process, and then ends up not just overweight but also tired and depressed. If Sharon had nothing else to do in the world besides take care of her body, she could probably keep her weight down with constant vigilance to exercise and diet. Women celebrities whose livelihood depends on staying slim often have a personal trainer for maintaining their exercise regimen and a personal cook to create tasty, healthful meals three times a day. Nice work if you can get it, but it would be a big mistake to feel guilty because you can't keep up. (And by the way, men past the age of thirty or so who are polled about everything from breast implants to weight gain admit that though they like to look at svelte, busty actresses, they actually prefer their real-life women the way they are, complete with saggy breasts and big hips. These polls don't often show up in women's magazines, because then what would they sell in their glossy pages?)

Sharon went to see Dr. Hanley, who worked with her over six months to balance her hormones and her blood sugar, support her overworked adrenal glands, and gradually shift herself and her family to a diet that would be nutritious and delicious without promoting weight gain. The new dietary regimen was a popular move with her husband, who was gaining weight around his midriff. Although Sharon didn't lose any weight in those first six months, she did stop gaining it. Once her energy was restored, she began gradually increasing her exercise by taking walks with her family, but she found that she preferred spending her "alone" time in her garden rather than at the gym. Over the next year Sharon lost about ten pounds and then remained steady. She was healthy in every way, had her energy back, and was very happy with the balance she had created in her life. And she had discovered that her husband didn't find her any less sexually desirable even though she had become heavier—in fact, he told her that her more rounded figure was sensual.

It is perfectly possible to weigh more than your doctor's charts say you should and be very healthy. As women age, they naturally put on weight, especially in their hips, thighs, buttocks, and abdomen. As we mentioned in an earlier chapter, in an ideal world this extra fat provides protection. As women age and ovarian production of estrogen declines, the fat cells produce estrogen. Your premenopausal years will be much happier if you stop worrying about your weight and put all that energy into more positive channels.

Another factor in premenopausal weight gain is eating to correct hormonal imbalances. It's quite natural to head for caffeine, sugar, and refined carbohydrates when your energy is low, in an attempt to pick it up again. A woman who feels tired, mentally foggy, or irritable will instinctively head for foods that stimulate the adrenals (caffeine), as well as increase glucose and serotonin levels in the brain (sugar and refined carbohydrates). Your brain is an extremely glucose-dependent organ, and serotonin is the same feel-good brain chemical that is increased by Prozac and similar drugs.

Once you are familiar with your body's signals and symptoms, you can be more conscious about how you re-gain balance when you're feeling out of sorts. You might choose consciously to use food to temporarily regain your balance, while also using natural hormones, nutri-tional supplements, and exercise to achieve long-term stability.

When we say that it's okay to gain some weight, of course we're not talking about obesity, which does in-crease your risk factors for just about every disease you can think of. There's a difference between putting on some weight as you age and being obese. If your health and ability to move around physically are compromised by your weight, then you can consider yourself obese. If this is the case, you are in an unhealthy state and you need to bring your body back into balance.

Estrogen is made and stored in fatty tissues, so obesity is a major cause of estrogen dominance, and vice versa. Estrogen causes weight gain by its action of converting food energy into stored energy called fat. That is why it is given to steers grown for slaughter. Since testosterone is an antagonist and opposes estrogen, calves are castrated and then given estrogen to promote rapid growth on less food.

Women who are estrogen dominant tend to retain water and crave simple carbohydrates like sugar, baked goods, and chips. Women who are obese also tend to become insulin resistant, which means sugar isn't being removed from the blood and utilized properly. This sets up imbalances in the adrenal glands and increases cortisol levels, which in turn affect the reproductive organs. Your body works as a unit—when one part of it is out of balance, the rest tends to follow.

Simply following the diet and lifestyle suggestions in chapters 13, 14, and 15 will help the majority of women maintain a reasonable weight through their menopausal years. We're not saying it's going to make you as slim and muscular as you were when you were twenty. That's not healthy or realistic. When you eat wholesome foods, balance your hormones, and get a little exercise, you feel better and your energy increases, which naturally allows excess weight to drop off. What's left is most likely what Mother Nature intended you to have to keep you healthy. If you look around you and notice that your sisters, cousins, aunts, and mothers are all around the same weight and they're healthy, just know you're in good company, along with the vast majority of women around the world, and relax.

❧ THYROID DYSFUNCTION

A woman named Hannah wrote Dr. Lee about her experience with low thyroid and hormone imbalance:

> Five years ago (I was 31) during my pregnancy, I began dealing with what I will call "hormonal

issues." After my son was born, I figured things would level out again, but when he was 7 months old the symptoms were not only still there, they were getting worse! One sobering realization really gnawed at me—no matter how much willpower and determination I had, I could not lose weight. I just continued to gain. This was in spite of doing all the commonsense things we're told to do—exercise, cut calories, and fat grams. Not until I gained an additional 20 pounds in one weekend and my neck swelled to the point of causing my gold chain to almost cut off my circulation did I admit to myself, "Something is really wrong here. I need help." And by the way, I'm embarrassed to admit that before this I thought that PMS and other hormonal complaints were an excuse to lose self-control.

Here is the list of symptoms I was ignoring: extreme fatigue, mood swings, water retention, breast swelling and tenderness, severe headaches, foggy thinking and inability to concentrate, joint pain, dry and cracking skin, vaginal dryness and odor, heavy dark menstrual flow and clotting, bleeding gums, poor night vision, and irritability (well, wouldn't you be irritable with all these symptoms—ha!).

I was afraid my ob-gyn would tell me I was losing it, but instead he told me that my thyroid was virtually inactive and gave me some Synthroid along with some vitamins and nutritional advice. This took care of a lot of the symptoms and I functioned well for a couple of years except for sinus infections. Then things got really strange. All my old symptoms returned and worse. I could no longer balance the checkbook, I was driving badly, my husband had to help me complete my sentences, and I couldn't even remember simple things like my own phone number. I had insomnia, hot flashes, severe headaches, and mood swings and such extreme fatigue that I couldn't take care of my family or even my own personal hygiene. I went to my doctor and he determined that my thyroid was fine, diagnosed me with having manic depression, or bipolar disorder, and prescribed me an antidepressant.

That's when I found your book, *What Your Doctor May* Not *Tell You about Menopause,* and, after reading it and recognizing myself, asked my doctor to check my hormone levels. He did and my progesterone was low. Since the night I began the cream, under his supervision, I've not had a single hot flash, I'm sleeping well again, and actually feel rested when I wake up. I'm off the antidepressant, I've lost two dress sizes and I no longer need a nap in the afternoon. I'm also taking supplements to help me clear the toxins from my body, calcium and magnesium, a multivitamin, the herb dong quai and a supplement for my allergies. I finally have a life again, and this situation has caused me and my husband to take more responsibility for our health.

During the first few years that Dr. Lee recommended progesterone cream to his menopausal patients, he noticed that those who were also taking thyroid medication often needed a reduced dose of it after a few months on the cream. Quite a number of these patients eventually were able to discontinue thyroid supplementation completely. When he went back and reviewed their cases he found that many of them had been started on thyroid supplements for symptoms of fatigue, weight gain, low basal body temperature, and other signs and symptoms often associated with low thyroid (hypothyroidism) in spite of normal thyroid tests.

After nearly twenty years of observing this phenomenon, Dr. Lee has come to believe that estrogen dominance interferes with or inhibits thyroid hormone activity, and progesterone facilitates thyroid hormone activity. Estrogen and thyroid do have some opposing actions. Estrogen instructs the body to store calorie intake as fat tissue, whereas thyroid increases the body's ability to metabolize fat for energy. Progesterone, on the other hand, has an anabolic action similar to that of thyroid: They both promote energy production and raise body temperature. Progesterone deficiency would lead to lower basal temperature, simulating symptoms of hypothyroidism. The most common symptoms of low thyroid (hypothyroidism) can include:

- Fatigue and weakness
- Low basal temperature (measured under the armpit first thing in the morning)

- Dry or coarse skin and hair
- Cold hands and feet
- Slurred or slow speech
- Poor memory
- Weight gain

There's no doubt that many premenopausal women are truly suffering from hypothyroidism. However, women who have symptoms of hypothyroidism but come out "normal" on a thyroid test may be progesterone deficient and can often be adequately treated by restoring normal progesterone levels using transdermal progesterone creams. This thyroid-balancing effect does not occur with the synthetic progestins such as Provera or the oral progesterone pills.

Dr. Hanley saw so many women in her practice with low thyroid function that she began digging deeper to find the causes, and she discovered that even small amounts of radiation can permanently destroy the thyroid gland. She found government statistics showing that in the 1950s the amount of radioactive fallout from nuclear weapons testing was enough to cause thyroid problems in an average person. Growing children exposed to the radiation were even more susceptible. Also, the ranges of normal used to determine thyroid function were calculated in the 1940s on twenty-two-year-old medical students, so she believes that they don't apply to premenopausal women. The consequence, Dr. Hanley believes, is an undiagnosed epidemic of low-level hypothyroidism.

If you have low thyroid symptoms, you can try using some progesterone cream for a few months. If you still have the symptoms, you can either use Armour Thyroid, which is a combination of cow (bovine) and pig (porcine) thyroid extract, or one of the synthesized thyroid hormones such as levothyroxine (Synthroid). There is much debate about which one of these forms of thyroid supplementation works best, but we believe the jury is still out on this question.

❧ CHRONIC FATIGUE

Mitochondria are intracellular organelles, tiny "power plants" within a cell's cytoplasm that supply the cell with energy. They convert the energy of chemical bonds of glucose and other nutrients into a substance called adenosine triphosphate (ATP) for energy use by the organism. Damage to the mitochondria can result in chronic fatigue. Our mitochondria have their own DNA, which is passed only from mother to child. Thus, damaged mitochrondia can be inherited.

In animals and humans, the mitochondria, in addition to producing ATP, also break down a few chemical bonds of the cholesterol molecule to produce pregnenolone, which is used by animals in the biosynthesis of progesterone and DHEA.

Efficient functioning of the mitochondria is blocked by estrogen, X radiation, ultraviolet (UV) radiation (usually from the sun), some unsaturated fatty acids, and iron, but it is facilitated by triodothyronine (or T_3, a form of thyroid hormone produced by your body), full-spectrum light, vitamin B2 (riboflavin), vitamins A and E, and copper. When estrogen interferes with efficient functioning of mitochondria, the result is not only less pregnenolone synthesis (and therefore less progesterone and DHEA) but also less energy for the body. This may be a factor in explaining progesterone deficiency in menstruating women: Mitochondrial damage interferes with the production of the precursor of progesterone.

The substance nicotinamide adenine dinucleotide (NADH) plays a pivotal role in the production of ATP, but until recently it was too unstable to take as a substance. Austrian biochemist Georg Birkmayer, M.D., Ph.D., discovered a way to stabilize NADH, which he has patented and made available as a supplement. In FDA-approved, double-blind placebo studies, NADH has been shown to significantly improve the symptoms of both Parkinson's disease and chronic fatigue. It's an expensive supplement, but if you're suffering from chronic fatigue that is due even in part to mitochondrial damage, NADH could help get you up and going again. NADH is available at most health food stores and must be taken on an empty stomach, preferably first thing in the morning. Follow the dosage instructions on the container.

❧ LOSS OF SEX DRIVE

"I'm forty-three years old and still having periods but I've lost interest in sex. What's wrong?" This is a common complaint heard in doctor's offices from premenopausal women. Libido is mistakenly thought by most doctors to come from estrogen, but excess estrogen can have the opposite effect, squelching libido with its side effects of water retention and irritability. The hormones that improve libido are progesterone and testosterone. From an evolutionary point of view this makes sense, since progesterone is the dominant hormone at ovulation, when a woman is most fertile.

Progesterone is usually the best hormone to start with to improve libido. Your doctor might recommend testosterone, but even slightly high levels can have masculinizing effects and can make libido more intense than most women might want. Dr. Lee likes to say that when progesterone levels are restored you won't become a sex maniac—the guy across the room will just become a little better looking.

Estrogen deficiency can cause vaginal dryness and atrophy, which can make sex painful. In that case, a little bit of vaginal estrogen cream (look for natural estriol) used a few times a week usually solves the problem.

❧ HAIR LOSS

When progesterone levels fall as a result of ovarian follicle failure (lack of ovulation), the body responds by increasing its production of the adrenal cortical steroid, androstenedione, an alternative precursor for the production of other adrenal cortical hormones and testosterone. Androstenedione conveys some androgenic (male-like) properties, in this case, male-pattern hair loss. When progesterone levels are raised by progesterone supplements, the androstenedione level will gradually fall, and your normal hair growth will eventually resume. Since hair growth is a slow process, it may take four to six months for the effects to become apparent.

Taking too much of the adrenal hormone DHEA or the hormone androstenedione can also cause hair loss in women. DHEA may be converted into androstenedione in the body, or it may carry its own androgenic effects.

❖ SKIN: ROSACEA, RASHES, DERMATITIS

Both Dr. Lee and Dr. Hanley have heard from many women whose skin problems cleared up after a few months of using progesterone cream. One woman wrote Dr. Lee and told him that her severe rosacea, which had given her a red nose and for which she had been prescribed cortisone drugs, had begun to clear up in a matter of days after starting to use progesterone cream.

❖ ENDOMETRIOSIS

Endometriosis is very difficult to treat and is one of the most painful afflictions a woman can endure. Though the cause is unknown, the symptoms of cramping and abdominal pain result from islets of endometrial (uterine) tissue that somehow migrate outside the uterus and are scattered throughout the pelvic area, attaching to the ovaries, the bladder wall, the intestinal walls, and membranes in the abdomen. The endometrial tissue responds to the monthly surges of estrogen by becoming blood filled, and at menstruation, when the uterine endometrium is shed, the endometrial islets also "shed" blood, but it has nowhere to go. The blood in the tissues creates local inflammation, which, in pelvic and abdominal tissues, is very painful.

We know that the symptoms of endometriosis pretty much disappear during pregnancy, only to flare up again after delivery. This suggests that the sex hormones are involved and, further, that the high progesterone levels of pregnancy may be the important factor.

Dr. Lee has successfully treated endometriosis using relatively high doses of progesterone cream to create a pseudopregnancy state from day 5 to day 28 (or whenever your normal cycle ends) of the menstrual month. This involves using 40 to 60 mg progesterone daily during these days, or 960 mg per month. This will often cause the pain to subside by the third or fourth month. In some patients with particularly stubborn endometriosis, he has increased the daily dose to 80 mg per day. Once the pain has been reduced, the dosage may be reduced gradually each month to find a dose that keeps the pain away.

Progesterone, at doses similar to the first month of pregnancy, limits the endometrial tissue buildup caused by estrogen. By preventing the monthly release of blood in the endometrial islets, the inflammation that previously flared each month will subside, and the healing forces of nature will return the endometrial islets back to normal tissue.

Dr. Hanley encourages women with endometriosis to take a few days off for rest each month when they first began menstruating. Most of these women have been forced to take time off because of their endometriosis, so she suggests they make it a choice and spend the time nurturing themselves. She has found that this alone can significantly reduce the pain. If you have endometriosis and it's not realistic for you to take a few days off, at the very least try to schedule in some nurturing time for yourself, even if it's just a bubble bath or going to bed early with a cup of hot tea and a good book.

❧ HEALING ENDOMETRIOSIS ❧

What to Do

- Take high doses (40–60 mg daily) of progesterone cream from day 5–28 (or whenever your normal cycle ends) of the menstrual cycle (please work in partnership with a health care professional when using high doses of any hormone or supplement).
- Use an herbal formula for endometriosis that includes some or all of the following herbs: licorice root, prickly ash, motherwort (*Leonurus cardiaca*), *Vitex*, wild yam (*Dioscorea*), cramp bark (*Viburnum opulus*).

What to Avoid

- Anything that creates estrogen dominance or high hormone levels (with the exception of progesterone)
- Birth control pills

❖ DEPRESSION, THE BRAIN, AND THE COPPER-ZINC CONNECTION

You might have noticed that the loss of zinc and the retention of copper are listed among the symptoms of estrogen dominance, but you may not be aware of the significance of these two minerals. Though our bodies need only very small amounts of zinc and copper, the need and the relative balance of them are very important. One of the most important functions of minerals is their role as a cofactor for enzymes.

Enzymes are special proteins made inside our cells from amino acids via instructions from our genes. They perform all the biochemical work of the cell: turning food into energy, building other important molecules, destroying toxins, utilizing oxygen, and creating all the material necessary for life. Each enzyme has a specific function and the function of each is enhanced by specific vitamin and mineral cofactors. Without the vitamin and mineral cofactors, the enzyme cannot do its work with efficiency.

In particular, copper and zinc are involved in enzymes

within brain cells. Some of these enzymes create the neurotransmitters that brain cells use to transmit their messages from one brain cell to another, whereas other enzymes inactivate neurotransmitters when they are no longer needed for brain cell transmissions. Proper balance is the key. The balance of zinc and copper is very important in the brain's regulation of mood and reaction to stress. Vitamin B_6 is the vitamin most commonly needed by these particular enzymes, which is why it often is effective in treating depression.

Estrogen has potent effects on the brain. That works to your advantage when it's in balance but to your disadvantage when it is present in excess or is not balanced by progesterone. For example, one brain enzyme, monoamine oxidase (MAO), can cause depression when it is elevated. Lower levels of MAO clear depression. Short-term estrogen elevation tends to inhibit MAO (thus preventing depression) whereas the progestins tend to elevate MAO (thus perhaps causing depression).

Dr. Ellen Grant has made an association between high copper levels, low zinc levels, and the rage that can be associated with PMS. Long-term exposure to excessive estrogen (and progestins) can lead to copper and zinc imbalance. Longer-term estrogen elevation tends to raise the blood levels of a protein, ceruloplasmin, which binds to copper and prevents it from getting into brain cells where it is needed for proper enzyme function. At the same time, the estrogen increases copper levels in the blood, which decreases zinc levels.

As blood levels of copper rise, more copper is lost in

sweat and hair. Brain cell copper is eventually depleted. Copper and zinc levels in blood tend to have an inverse relation. Higher blood copper levels deplete brain cell copper stores and cause reduced blood zinc levels. Imbalance of these two minerals results in unbalanced activity of the enzymes for which they are cofactors and leads to exaggerated stress reactions, serious mood swings, and depression. Sound familiar?

Restoring normal copper and zinc levels is a bit tricky. As noted above, higher serum levels of ceruloplasmin raised blood levels of copper but depleted brain cell levels. If you withhold supplemental copper, the brain cell problem gets worse. If you add copper, you further depress zinc levels, and zinc-dependent enzymes cannot work effectively. The goal, of course, is to restore normal balance of these two important minerals.

To complicate matters, blood serum tests do not accurately reflect cellular levels of these minerals. (Serum is the watery, noncellular portion of blood.) The answer is to measure copper and zinc levels within cells carried by the blood, such as red blood cells and white blood cells. The cellular levels of these minerals are controlled by the cell membrane. A healthy cell membrane allows just the right amount of potassium, magnesium, copper, and zinc to be kept within the cell while at the same time keeping out sodium that would result in water influx and intracellular edema. Estrogen and the progestins impair this action of the cell membrane whereas natural progesterone restores proper function of it. If hormone balance is achieved and your diet contains healthy amounts of fresh, unprocessed foods, the mineral imbalance corrects itself.

✤ PREVENTING OSTEOPOROSIS

You probably think that osteoporosis is a disease of thin bones suffered by little old ladies with dowager's humps. Or maybe you think it's a calcium deficiency disease. In truth, osteoporosis is a progressive disease with many factors contributing to its cause. It is a disease of excessive bone loss and decreased bone density; that is, over time there is less bone and what is left is lighter and more porous. The danger in osteoporosis is an increased risk of bone fractures that can be painful and debilitating enough to lead to premature death.

If you're over the age of thirty-five, your bone loss has very likely already begun. Bone loss begins long before menopause and can be accelerated by a chronic loss of progesterone due to anovulatory cycles. Estrogen plays the role of slowing bone loss, but it is progesterone that plays the lead role in building bone. Even with high doses of estrogen, if you're not making new bone rapidly enough to replace old bone, you will eventually get osteoporosis.

As the typical American woman approaches menopause, osteoporosis is already under way, and she will lose 20 percent or more of her bone mass *before* menopause. When progesterone deficiency is suspected (by symptoms of relative estrogen dominance), osteoporosis can be not only prevented but also reversed by the addition of progesterone along with a program of proper diet, modest supplements of important vitamins and minerals, and some exercise. The bone benefits of progesterone require only 15 to 20 mg per day of transdermal progesterone. In premenopausal women, the dosage period is from day 12 to day 26 of the menstrual month. (See chapter 16 for details.)

If you are at risk for osteoporosis, we strongly recommend that you read the detailed chapter on osteoporosis in Dr. Lee's book, *What Your Doctor May* Not *Tell You about Menopause,* and start your personal prevention program now. Women most at risk for osteoporosis have a close relative who has it; are Caucasian; thin and petite; don't exercise; smoke; have a poor diet; and use antacids, diuretics, sleeping pills, and/or cortisone drugs regularly.

Chapter 11

❧

The Dangers of Hormonal Contraceptives

*D*octors tend to be very reluctant *not* to prescribe birth control pills to a young, sexually active woman. Because diaphragms and condoms are somewhat less effective at preventing pregnancy (and more prone to be used incorrectly), and because they are considered more awkward and less convenient to use, doctors fear that not using the Pill means a woman will get pregnant. Sitting face-to-face with a woman who has a bright future ahead of her, the doctor has a choice between a possible abortion or unwanted child, or giving a prescription for a birth control pill. This is a very difficult choice to make. There's no doubt whatsoever that birth control pills, shots, or implants are a very effective, trouble-free form of birth control, but it is also clear that they are very dangerous.

Every doctor—and patient—who is torn by this decision should be required to read Dr. Ellen Grant's *The Bitter Pill: How Safe Is the Perfect Contraceptive?* This searing indictment of the Pill is written by a British doctor who was hired in the early 1960s to work in a London clinic and test varying combinations and dosages of birth control pills. She took the job full of optimism and idealism, believing that birth control pills were the answer to overpopulation and that they represented a new kind of freedom for women. But as the months and the years went by, Dr. Grant saw serious, often life-threatening side effects occur with all dosages and combinations of the pills, which comprised varying dosages of synthetic progestins (called progestogens in the United Kingdom) and estrogens. Changing the dosage or the type of the synthetic hormone merely substituted one set of symptoms for another. Today the claim is that lower dose birth control pills cause fewer symptoms and are less dangerous, but there is no hard evidence that this is true.

Even in a clinic where her sole purpose was to work with women taking birth control pills and make assessments as to how they were working, Dr. Grant noticed that she wasn't being officially required to ask in any detail about side effects. The major concern of those testing the birth control pills were (1) did it prevent pregnancy, and (2) were the immediate side effects reduced enough so that women would keep taking the pills? There was no long-term follow-up, nor was there any genuine concern for possible long-term consequences of taking the pill. The justification in the minds of those manufacturing and testing the pills was that the benefit to humanity as a whole of a lower birth rate outweighed the risks and negative side effects to individual women.

After a decade of working with oral contraceptives, Dr. Grant decided that they were so dangerous that nobody should take them and she began to speak out against them. Predictably, nobody in mainstream medicine wanted to listen. It is unfortunate that her book is out of print, but you may be able to find it at a used bookstore or through Amazon Books' Web site: www.amazon.com. The following list of side effects were among those that Dr. Grant consistently noticed in women taking all combinations of birth control pills.

- Six times greater risk of thrombosis (blood clot in a blood vessel)
- Four times greater risk of dying from a stroke (blood clot or broken blood vessel in the brain)
- Four times the risk of heart attack
- Three times greater risk of headaches
- Double the risk of migraine headaches
- Double the risk of high blood pressure
- Double the risk of death from an accident or violence
- Double the risk of dying from cancer, especially cervical, breast, and endometrial cancer, in women 25 to 50 years old
- Increased risk of ovarian cancer
- Increased cancer risk in smokers, especially melanoma and lung cancer

- More thyroid and liver cancers
- Altered immune function
- Reduction of antioxidant levels, especially in the liver
- A higher rate of birth defects and birthmarks in the children of women who have used oral contraceptives
- Increased risk of osteoporosis caused by blood vessel abnormalities in the bone
- Increased risk of ovarian cysts, infections, urinary tract problems, cervical erosion (dysplasia), allergies, gall-bladder disease, sinus infections, ulcerative colitis, Crohn's disease, lung disease, epilepsy, loss of libido, infertility, pituitary tumors, and schizophrenia
- Higher rates of antianxiety drug, antidepressant, or sleeping pill usage
- Higher likelihood of having their uterus and/or ovaries removed

All of this takes into account the fact that only the healthiest women were included in the studies, that those who dropped out within a few months were excluded from most of the studies, and that deaths were frequently attributed to preexisting causes. Dr. Grant's very specific accounts of how statistics have been juggled to make the Pill seem safer are chilling, particularly in hiding the fact that taking an oral contraceptive clearly creates an increased risk of breast cancer.

It is a tragedy in the making that the use of hormone "shots" (i.e., Depo-Provera) has recently become trendy among young women, and doctors are willingly giving them. It seems like an easy solution to birth control—

you don't even have to remember to take a pill—but the consequences can be just as devastating as taking oral contraceptives. The difference is that the potential toxicity is much greater, and you're stuck with a three-month supply of hormones in your body, which you can't stop if you have immediate side effects.

Oral contraceptives also affect nutrient levels. Women who use synthetic hormonal contraceptives tend to be deficient in vitamin B6 (pyridoxine), folic acid, vitamin B12, vitamin B2 (riboflavin), and the important antioxidant beta carotene. These synthetic hormones also put significant additional stress on the liver, lowering levels of the important antioxidant glutathione, which in turn puts the liver at greater risk from liver-damaging toxins such as prescription drugs and over-the-counter drugs such as acetaminophen (Tylenol), and pesticides.

Serotonin is well known these days as a brain chemical made from the amino acid tryptophan, which helps regulate mood. A serotonin deficiency can cause depression. Although estrogens can raise serotonin levels, according to Dr. Grant, oral contraceptives containing progestins interfere with serotonin production, and this may be part of the reason that they cause depression in so many women.

Other nutrients that can be depleted by the use of oral contraceptives include magnesium and manganese.

❧ OTHER BIRTH CONTROL OPTIONS

There aren't any ideal birth control options that combine a high rate of preventing pregnancy with ease of use. Synthetic hormone contraceptives (birth control pills, shots, and implants) are clearly very dangerous, as is the IUD, which creates a constant state of irritation in the uterus. The spermicides used with diaphragms, cervical caps, and condoms have their own set of problems. Although they may be safer than the Pill, the same qualities that make them toxic to sperm also make them toxic to you!

An approach to preventing pregnancy that is very safe and effective when used properly is called the ovulation method (you may have also heard it referred to as the rhythm method), which was first clearly spelled out in a book by Evelyn and John Billings some twenty years ago. They were Catholics who wanted to be responsible about having children and space them apart, while at the same time observing the rules of the Church governing birth control. The ovulation method involves tracking your menstrual cycles, your body temperature, and the consistency of your vaginal mucus so that you know the days when you're fertile. On those days you either abstain from having intercourse or you use an alternate form of protection. This method, pooh-poohed by most physicians, is actually as effective as condoms and diaphragms when it is used conscientiously. It is an approach that both honors your body and its natural cycles and increases your awareness of those cycles. In the book *The*

New Our Bodies, Ourselves, the Boston Women's Health Book Collective gives fairly detailed information about the ovulation method as well as resources for finding more information.

Chapter 12

— ❧ —

The Relationship of Hormones to Breast Cancer and Other Women's Cancers

Dr. Lee receives dozens of letters every week from women with questions about hormones. One of the most touching letters he received was from a woman named Sally who had been given a diagnosis of breast cancer two-and-a-half years prior to writing him. Just a few months before she was diagnosed, a friend of hers had finally died after a difficult battle with breast cancer. Sally had watched her friend dutifully follow the instructions of her physicians to the letter. She went through the agonies of a lumpectomy, chemotherapy, and radiation, only to have the breast cancer show up just over a year later in her other breast and her lungs; she died nine months later.

Sally was determined that she wasn't going to take the same path. She had a lumpectomy but chose not to have chemotherapy and radiation treatments because her doctors couldn't show her any evidence that those treatments would increase her chances of survival. She began to explore alternatives. After much research, she decided to work with a naturopathic doctor who recommended a very demanding course of fasting and cleansing followed by significant diet changes, nutritional supplements, counseling, support groups, and a natural progesterone cream. At first, Sally had agreed to everything except the progesterone, because she had heard so much conflicting information about it. The naturopath recommended she read Dr. Lee's book, *What Your Doctor May* Not *Tell You about Menopause,* which she did, and she then felt she had the facts she needed to make the decision to use the progesterone.

A year after her initial diagnosis, and closely following the advice of the naturopath, Sally was diagnosed as cancer-free. She was writing to say that she had just had another series of tests and that she remained cancer-free, and she thanked him for the information in the book. She wrote that she was sad that her friend who died hadn't had the benefit of alternative therapies.

The information in this chapter about hormones and cancer is very new and controversial. Women who opt for alternative treatments to radiation, chemotherapy, and tamoxifen should be prepared to take them very seriously, to make dramatic lifestyle changes, and to devote a lot of time and energy to maintaining these changes.

Treating any kind of cancer is a life-and-death battle that demands focused attention and the willingness to change the conditions that created the disease in the first place.

❖ SOME CANCER BASICS

Cancer occurs when cells multiply (proliferate) faster than normal, lose differentiation, and have slowed apoptosis (programmed cell death) rates. This is usually caused by damage or some sort of toxic environment within the cell sufficient to affect the cell's chromosomes (the structures in the nucleus that hold genetic information). Such damage can result from viruses, radiation, genetic predisposition, or exposure to toxic chemicals.

The cell is usually protected against cancer by a variety of defenses, all relying on proper nutrition, proper hormone balance, and proper enzyme function. Lacking these, the cell cannot neutralize and/or excrete toxic products and cannot repair itself well enough to counter the damage of the factors above. When sufficient gene damage occurs, the cell reverts to a more primitive life form and becomes a cancer cell. Since the chance of irreparable genetic damage increases over time, the chance of developing cancer increases with age.

The human body contains approximately 64 trillion cells. A drop of blood contains about 3,000 to 5,000 white blood cells and 5 million red blood cells. If a single cell in one's breast becomes a cancer cell, it usually takes 8 to 12 years for that cell to multiply into a detectable mass. Another way of understanding the rate at which breast cancer tumors grow is that they double in size every three to four months.

When first detectable by mammogram, it takes only a year or two for a breast cancer tumor to increase in size to be detectable by hand palpation. This two-year time interval has little effect on the likelihood of a breast cancer to metastasize (spread through the lymph or blood system to other parts of the body). This is why mammography has little effect on ultimate mortality from breast cancer. Both Dr. Lee and Dr. Hanley believe that the jury is still very much out on the benefit of mammography and that women can probably achieve the same benefit by carefully examining their own breasts once a month.

It is now recognized that surgery, radiation, and chemotherapy are less than satisfactory in treating breast cancer. If we are to minimize the scourge of breast cancer, we must learn to identify and limit the causative or cancer-promoting factors and maximize the protective or cancer-preventative factors. In this regard, it is sobering to realize that only 5 percent of the National Cancer Institute's budget is allocated to research on cancer prevention.

❖ USE THE AMAS TEST BEFORE INVASIVE SURGERY

Testing for the presence of cancer hasn't been very effective in the past. Although increases in some types of immune cells can be a generic indicator of a potential cancer, specific tests such as pap smears and prostate cancer tests are notoriously inaccurate. At long last, a new test has provided us with an accurate method for detecting a malignant cancer. After nearly twenty-five years of research and testing, a Harvard-trained scientist named Dr. Samuel Bogoch and his wife, Dr. Eleanor Bogoch, have created a generic blood test for all types of cancer that will detect any type of malignancy, however small, anywhere in the body. The test has an accuracy rate of 95 percent, and 99 percent on the second test. The test is called AMAS, or antimalignan antibody in serum. It is patented, and has been approved by the FDA after extensive testing.

What the Bogoch team discovered is that cancer cells release a substance called malignan, immediately recognized by the immune system, which responds with antibodies to destroy it. These antibodies, called antimalignans, can be detected by the AMAS test.

The AMAS test has three important applications. One is as a part of an annual checkup. If the AMAS test is normal, other more invasive or inaccurate diagnostic tools don't need to be used. The second is to monitor whether a cancer has been cured. After treatment of a malignant cancer, the AMAS will prove definitively whether the malignancy is gone. The third application, after other diagnostic tests (such as an X ray or mammogram) have indicated a possible cancer, allows the AMAS to confirm whether it is malignant, avoiding an invasive biopsy.

If you have a high cancer risk (you have one or more

people in your immediate family who have had it), an annual AMAS test, beginning in your mid-thirties, can give you the early warning that can lead to early detection, particularly with breast and ovarian cancers because they can be difficult to detect until they are advanced. (See Resources for details.)

❧ BREAST CANCER BASICS

Since 1950 breast cancer incidence has risen by 60 percent. Some will argue that this is due to better and earlier detection. However, for women over eighty years of age, the incidence of breast cancer has risen in the past thirty years from one of 30 women to one of 8 women.

In any given breast cancer tumor, not all cells are identical. Cells within any given tumor show obvious differences. Present anticancer treatments may destroy or negate some but not all of the cancer cells. This is the reason it is unlikely that our present treatments will improve our cure rates.

Like all cancers, breast cancer cells are not foreign invaders but, as British researcher A. B. Astrow aptly put it, "Essentially normal cells in which proportionately small changes in their genes lead to large changes in behavior." We do not know much about the causes or the factors that change a normal cell into a cancer cell, but important new research is pointing the way.

❧ PROGRAMMED CELL DEATH GIVES US NEW LIFE

One of the most important new findings has to do with apoptosis (ah-po-'toe-sis), or programmed cell death. With the exception of neural and muscle cells, all the cells of the body are constantly being replaced with newly made cells. This requires that previously made cells normally live for a specified period of time and then die as new cells come along to replace them. The death of old cells is necessary for continued good health. Old skin cells are shed, as are the lining cells of respiratory organs and the gastrointestinal system. In the breast, however, the old cells that undergo apoptosis are consumed by macrophages (special white blood cells). It is now well understood by cancer specialists that delayed apoptosis of older cells increases their risk of becoming cancer cells.

Apoptosis literally means "falling away" like leaves from a tree in the autumn. It is often explained as "programmed cell suicide." The point is that good health demands that older cells must die off as new cells are continually being created.

❧ CELL DIFFERENTIATION AND PROLIFERATION

Breast cancer originates as a change in milk duct epithelial cells and, as with other types of cancers, in addition to a slowing of apoptosis, these cells show a *loss of differentiation* and *increased proliferation rate* compared with normal breast cells. As cells grow, they differentiate into the special type of tissue they were meant to be. Usually, those that are proliferating or multiplying faster will also be less differentiated. The more differentiated the cell, the slower it will proliferate and the more it will be like a normal cell (and therefore less threatening).

We know a great deal about factors that promote growth of cancer cells once they come into existence. This is important since the faster the growth rate, the less time it takes to become life threatening. A comparison of breast cancer with prostate cancer is enlightening. In a man over sixty-five years of age, prostate cancer has a doubling time of five years; in a woman with breast cancer, the doubling time may be as short as three months. Obviously, slowing the proliferation rate would be advantageous to one's survival time. In this regard, we find that estrogen increases proliferation rate of breast epithelial cells, while progesterone slows it down considerably. We will discuss this in more detail shortly.

When comparing the hormone receptors of breast cancer cells with the state of differentiation, it is found that a predominance of estrogen receptors correlates with less-differentiated, more dangerous cancer cells; the presence of progesterone receptors, on the other hand, correlates with cancer cells that are more differentiated and less dangerous. Estrogen also activates an oncogene (cancer-promoting gene) called Bcl-2, which slows apoptosis. Progesterone activates gene p53, which restores proper apoptosis.

Thus, by considering apoptosis, cell differentiation,

and cell proliferation, we see that estrogen is a potent promoter of breast cancer whereas progesterone protects against breast cancer.

❧ EVIDENCE THAT PROGESTERONE IS PROTECTIVE

Dr. Lee has researched and networked with other scientists and clinicians extensively on the subject of breast cancer, and together they have arrived at some fascinating and valuable insights into this deadly disease. Dr. Lee has tried to approach the information with the question "What evidence would be persuasive, to both a woman and her physician, that progesterone is protective against breast cancer?"

One good way to test progesterone's effect on breast cancer incidence would be to measure estrogen and progesterone levels in a large number of women and follow their lives to observe any correlation in the subsequent incidence of breast cancer. This has been done. In 1981 L. D. Cowan and colleagues at Johns Hopkins, published their results showing that the breast cancer incidence was 5.4 times greater in women with low progesterone than in women who had good progesterone levels. This difference remained true despite any differences in age of menarche, age of menopause, history of oral contraceptive use, history of benign breast disease, or age of first birth of a child. Furthermore, when the incidence of all types of cancer was looked at, they found that the incidence was 10-fold higher in women with low progesterone levels compared to women with good progesterone levels.

What about progesterone levels in women at the time of breast cancer diagnosis? This too has been investigated. Breast cancer researcher Dr. David Zava tested estrogen and progesterone levels in breast tissue specimens from several thousand women who had undergone breast cancer surgery. Almost universally, they revealed a relative deficiency in progesterone relative to estrogen.

Does survival after breast cancer surgery differ in women with differing progesterone levels? At least ten retrospective studies demonstrate a longer disease-free or overall survival advantage in women who have breast cancer surgery in the early luteal phase of the menstrual cycle when progesterone is presumed to be at its highest levels compared with surgery performed during the proliferative phase when progesterone is very low.

Dr. William Hrushesky of the Stratton VA Medical Center in Albany, New York, reviewed these data in the *Journal of Women's Health* in 1996 and listed seven known mechanisms of action by which we can directly or indirectly conclude that progesterone inhibits breast cancer cell growth and/or metastases.

1. Cellular immunity (natural killer cell activity and interleukin-2) is compromised by unopposed estrogen and promoted by adequate progesterone.
2. DNA synthesis, cell proliferation, apoptosis, and tissue remodeling are modulated by these two hormones. Specifically, cell proliferation and delayed or

inhibited apoptosis are characteristics that promote cancer. Estradiol increases these actions, whereas progesterone decreases them.

3. Sex steroid receptors are rhythmically affected by the menstrual cycle. The luteal phase offers the more desirable time for breast cancer surgery since progesterone receptors tend to be highest at that time of the cycle.

4. Surgical trauma is associated with a modulation of the capacity of metastatic tumor cells both to bind estrogen and to divide. Surgical trauma activates dormant metastases. Doing this at a time of estrogen dominance is counterproductive to survival.

5. Blood vessel formation (angiogenesis), arrest, and destruction in the endometrial lining of the uterus are coordinated by the menstrual cycle. Angiogenesis favors tumor formation and is most active during the estrogen-rich, progesterone-poor early follicular phase of the cycle. Blood vessel formation is abruptly inhibited as vascularization in the ovarian follicle is completed and, at ovulation, the corpus luteum rapidly secretes increasing amounts of progesterone. Angiogenesis inhibition suppresses tumor cell growth because it cuts off the blood supply that feeds the tumor.

6. Vascular (blood vessel) permeability is a factor of cancer cell metastasis (spread). Here again, progesterone reduces vascular permeability and thus protects against cancer cell metastasis.

7. Circulating cancer cell clumps in the blood are more likely to increase chances that a cancer will spread.

The tendency of blood cells to clump changes rhythmically as a function of menstrual phases. The follicular phase, which occurs when progesterone is low and estrogen is high, is associated with increased platelet aggregability (more cell clumping and more strokes in estrogen-dominant women), higher concentration of fibrinogen (correlated with increased incidence of heart attacks), and less filterable, stiffer red blood cells (poor flow through capillaries). It is likely that estrogen dominance of the follicular phase also increases the aggregability of metastasizing cancer cells, thus increasing their metastatic efficiency.

In a 20-year study published in 1996 in the *British Journal of Cancer,* Dr. P. E. Mohr and colleagues reported that women with higher progesterone levels at the time of their breast cancer surgery had a significantly better survival rate at 18 years than those with a lower serum level of progesterone. Among women with good progesterone levels at the time of surgery, approximately 65 percent were surviving 18 years later, whereas among women with low progesterone levels at the time of surgery, only about 35 percent of the women were surviving (see figures 12.1 and 12.2).

❧ FACTS AND FIGURES ON WOMEN AND BREAST CANCER

Women of nonindustralized or less-industrialized countries have less breast cancer than women of the industrial-

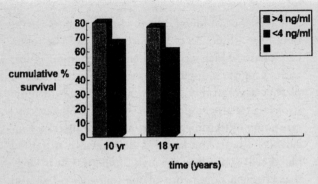

Figure 12.1. Overall Survival of Patients Based on Progesterone Levels
Cumulative percent survival at 10 and 18 years after breast cancer surgery in 92 women with greater than 4 ng/ml, compared to 197 women with less than 4 ng/ml. When comparing survival in node-positive patients, the difference is even greater.

Data from the Mohr study, British Journal of Cancer, *1996.*

ized countries. Dr. Peter Ellison of Harvard, using saliva hormone assay for World Health Organization (WHO) studies worldwide, has documented markedly higher estrogen levels among women of industrialized countries. Dr. Ellison is convinced that something in industrialized countries causes elevated estrogen levels and, therefore, a higher risk of breast cancer. He believes the elevated estrogen levels are due to excess calorie intake and lower expenditure of physical energy among women of industrialized countries. Regardless of cause, the fact re-

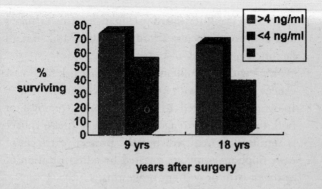

Figure 12.2. Overall Survival of Node-Positive Patients

Cumulative percent survival at 9 and 18 years after breast surgery in 47 node-positive patients with greater than 4 ng/ml serum progesterone compared with 93 node-positive patients with less than 4 ng/ml serum progesterone at the time of surgery.
Data from the Mohr study, British Journal of Cancer, *1996.*

mains that estrogen dominance correlates with higher incidence of breast cancer.

We also know some other pertinent information about breast cancer.

- Pregnancy occurring before age 30 is known to have a protective effect. Progesterone is the dominant hormone during pregnancy. Only the first full-term, early pregnancy conveys protection. Women having their first pregnancies before age 18 have approximately one-third the risk of women bearing the first child after age 35. Interrupted pregnancies (miscarriages and abortions) do not afford protection and may in fact increase the risk of breast cancer.

- Women without children are at a higher risk for breast cancer than those with one or more children.

- In women subjected to oophorectomy (removal of both ovaries) prior to age 40, the risk of breast cancer is significantly reduced, but the protective effects of early oophorectomy are negated by administration of estrogen with or without progestins.

- Treatment of men with estrogen (for prostatic cancer or after transsexual surgery) is associated with an increased risk of breast cancer.

- The most common age for the initial stages of breast or uterine cancer to be detected is five years or more *before* menopause. That is well before estrogen levels fall but coincides with a drop in progesterone.

❧ HOW SEX HORMONES INFLUENCE BREAST CELLS

To review the cancer basics, we know that there are three characteristics by which cancer cells differ from normal cells. They multiply, or proliferate, more rapidly, they are less differentiated (more immature) than normal cells, and they don't die (apoptosis) when they're supposed to. In contrast, a healthy cell multiples at normal rate, it differentiates into a specific type of cell, and it dies on a genetically predetermined schedule to make room for new cells.

It should not be surprising that sex hormones have a role in all three of these processes in breast cells. Women's breasts change at puberty when estrogen and progesterone production rises. The action of estradiol and progesterone on cell multiplication (proliferation) in breast cells was beautifully demonstrated in an important 1995 study by K. J. Chang and colleagues. It tested the effects of transdermal (via the skin) hormone applications on human breast milk duct epithelial cells, from which cancer is known to rise, in healthy young women planning to undergo minor breast surgery for benign breast disease (see figure 12.3).

In this study, the women were divided into the following four groups and began using one of the creams on their breasts 8 to 10 days before breast surgery.

Group A applied estradiol cream (1.5 mg) daily.
Group B applied progesterone cream (25 mg) daily.
Group C applied a combination of estradiol and progesterone (half doses each) daily.
Group D applied a placebo cream.

At surgery, biopsies were obtained for measuring estradiol and progesterone concentrations, and for tests of cell proliferation rates. In addition, blood plasma hormone levels were measured. The results indicated that estradiol cream increased estradiol concentration in breast cells by more than 100 percent and that the progesterone cream increased progesterone concentration in breast cells by 100 percent compared to the placebo

Figure 12.3. Effect of Hormones on Cell Division in Breast Tissue

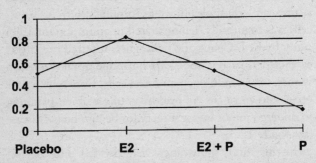

Effect of ten days of transdermal estradiol (E2 1.5 mg/day), estradiol plus progesterone (E2 +P), or progesterone (P 25 mg/day) on cell division compared with placebo.

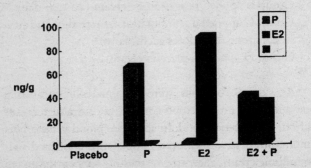

Effect of transdermal progesterone (P) and estradiol (E2) on breast cell hormone concentration.

Data from the Chang study.

cream. The combination cream resulted in a 50 percent increase of both hormones in breast cells. These findings clearly demonstrate that both hormones are well absorbed transdermally and accumulate in target tissues in the same manner as endogenous hormones.

The effect of these hormones on cell proliferation rates was equally clear. Estradiol increased cell proliferation rate by 230 percent whereas progesterone decreased it by more than 400 percent. The estradiol-progesterone combination cream maintained the normal proliferation rate. Again, this is clear evidence that unopposed estradiol stimulates hyperproliferation of breast epithelial cells and progesterone protects against this.

The fact that progesterone levels rose dramatically in breast cells proves that progesterone is well absorbed when applied to the skin. However, the blood plasma tests showed no measurable increase of progesterone concentration. This is an excellent illustration of the fact that bioavailable progesterone is carried in blood but not in blood plasma. This simple fact nullifies all previous claims based on plasma or serum testing that progesterone is not well absorbed through the skin.

This double-blind, randomized, placebo-controlled in vivo study proves that both estradiol and progesterone are well absorbed transdermally, and that estradiol stimulates proliferation of breast epithelial cells whereas progesterone reduces it. Since excessive cell proliferation (hyperplasia) is a recognized hallmark of potential cancer development, this study strongly suggests that estradiol increases that risk and progesterone protects against it.

Further, this study illustrates that plasma levels do not adequately reflect transdermal progesterone absorption. We now know that saliva hormone assay is far superior to "blood tests" in this matter. (See chapter 16 for details on transdermal progesterone and saliva testing.)

❧ THE RELATIONSHIP OF SEX HORMONES TO BREAST CANCER

Much confusion reigns in the understanding (or misunderstanding) of the relationship of sex hormones to breast cancer. Most experienced clinicians understand very well that estrogen is a promoter of breast cancer, and they also understand that progesterone balances or opposes undesirable side effects of estrogen. For reasons that are not entirely clear, conventional medicine has ignored the cancer-protective effects of progesterone in treating breast cancer despite many studies that offer solid evidence.

Even though a progestin is used in HRT to offset or oppose the cancer-promoting role of estrogen in endometrial cancer, progesterone has not been widely recognized for its similar role in breast cancer. Yet there are studies that clearly establish this relationship. As long ago as 1966, H. P. Leis reported treating 158 menopausal women (11 percent had a strong family history of breast cancer) with both estrogen and progesterone therapy for up to 14 years and none of the patients developed breast cancer.

In rodent studies by A. Inoh and colleagues, the protective effect of progesterone or tamoxifen was investigated in estrogen-induced mammary cancer. The ovaries of the rats were removed. Rats given estradiol had a high rate of mammary cancer. However, if tamoxifen or progesterone was given simultaneously with the estradiol, fewer tumors appeared, and the ones that did were smaller and less likely to spread. Tamoxifen, a patented drug, has been introduced as a standard treatment in conventional medicine, but progesterone has been ignored. Given the toxicity of tamoxifen, it is a tragedy that progesterone has been ignored in this context.

Although it's clear that genes play an important role in the predisposition to get breast cancer, an interesting study from London provides evidence that environmental influences are equally important. A comparison of breast cancer incidence in same-sex twins, both identical and fraternal, was made by researchers at the London School of Hygiene and Tropical Medicine. They found that a woman under age 45 with a twin sister who has breast cancer faces roughly eight times the average risk of getting the disease. The incidence of cancer greatly exceeded the risk faced by the general population. Further, the onset of cancer at a young age in one twin increased the chance that the other twin would develop the disease.

The fact that the increased cancer risk occurred in both fraternal and same-sex twins strongly suggests that the observed cancer proclivity was likely to involve a common prenatal environment rather than identical genes. This is quite similar to the adverse results in bird, fish, reptile, and mammal offspring of wildlife populations exposed to petrochemical xenoestrogens.

Further, there is a probable connection between breast cancer and elevated estrogen levels during pregnancy. Breast cancer, for instance, has been related to high birth weight, which, in turn, is related to high concentrations of estrogen in the womb. Women pregnant with twins have high concentrations of estrogen, presumably because of the much higher total birth weight of twins.

The scientific evidence is becoming ever more clear that prenatal exposure to estrogen dominance and/or petrochemical toxins can have deleterious effects that develop in later years of age. Given the important implications of these findings, it is in our best interest that research be drastically increased in this area.

❖ GETTING DOWN TO THE GENE LEVEL

Even more fundamental research now exists to link estrogen dominance to breast cancer. This new research involves genes.

If genes are damaged, for example, by radiation, toxins, or viruses, normal cells can develop into cancer cells. Certain genes called *proto-oncogenes* are normal to cells but may mutate into oncogenes with products that allow excessive proliferation or delayed apoptosis, resulting in the change of the cell into a cancer cell. Other genes, known to be tumor suppressor genes, inhibit cell division or stimulate apoptosis, thus preventing cancer. One's risk of cancer depends in large part on the relative activity of oncogenes versus tumor suppressor genes.

Several groups of molecular biologists have been investigating the actions of two genes named Bcl-2 and p53. Bcl-2 is the name of a proto-oncogene. Gene p53 is the name of a tumor suppressor gene. It is now well established that Bcl-2 production inhibits apoptosis and thereby promotes breast, ovary, endometrial, prostate cancer, and follicular B cell lymphoma. Conversely, up-regulation of p53 will inhibit Bcl-2 action, halt cell proliferation, and induce apoptosis, thus helping prevent cancer.

In cancer cell cultures, researchers B. Formby and T. S. Wiley found that when estradiol (in concentrations similar to what the human body makes) is added to the culture, Bcl-2 is activated and cancer growth is promoted. But the addition of progesterone (again in concentrations consistent with normal bodily levels) down-regulates Bcl-2 and up-regulates p53, thereby stopping cancer growth. This may sound simple, but it is actually a very profound and important piece of the cancer puzzle that is still being overlooked by mainstream medicine.

Thus, we now know at least one gene-related mechanism of action that connects estradiol to cancer promotion. Corroboration of these findings comes from research showing that one of the pathways of metabolizing estradiol and estrone leads to a by-product called estrogen-3,4-quinone that causes gene mutation and cancer. Let's look more closely at this work.

❧ THE DEEPER LEVELS OF HOW ESTROGEN CAUSES CANCER

Estrogen causes cancer at the gene level by the action of a certain metabolite (by-product) of estrone or estradiol in mutating critical genes: oncogenes and tumor suppressor genes. Dr. Ercole Cavalieri and his associates at the Eppley Institute for Research in Cancer, University of Nebraska Medical Center, have been working for thirty years on finding this answer. Through meticulous and extremely complex biochemical sleuthing, they have tracked the metabolism of estrogens through several pathways. They found that most of the pathways lead to harmless methylated products for excretion. However, one pathway leads to a metabolite, catechol estrogen-3,4-quinone, and this product not only binds to DNA, as some other estrogen metabolites do, but also uniquely alters gene proteins to cause carcinogenic mutations. This is the proverbial smoking gun. Figure 12.4 illustrates this mechanism.

❧ NATURAL DEFENSES AGAINST CANCER: AVOID JUNK FOOD AND EAT YOUR BROCCOLI

Mother Nature has created a series of defenses against the steps that lead estrogen to its carcinogenic metabolite. For example, the first step in this harmful pathway can be prevented if your diet is sufficient in the proper fatty acids (olive oil, and the naturally occurring oils found in

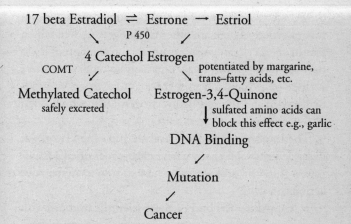

Figure 12.4. Angels of Life, Angels of Death: The Role of Estrogen in Cancer
Dr. Ercole Cavalieri, recalling that estrogen is necessary for the earliest critical stages of embryo life, and now recognizing the fatal consequences of estrogen metabolism following this pathway, refers to estrogens as the angels of life and the angels of death.

fish as well as in small amounts in fresh vegetables, whole grains, nuts, seeds, and fruits) rather than the synthetic trans–fatty acids (hydrogenated oils such as margarine) now so prevalent in the U.S. diet.

The second step can be blocked by sulfur-containing amino acids such as cysteine and methionine, found in garlic; onions; cruciferous vegetables such as broccoli and cauliflower; and beans. A deficiency of these sulfated amino acids allows the metabolic progression to the carcinogenic gene mutation.

We now see that estrone and estradiol are true initiators of cancer. There are other carcinogens as well which stimulate, accelerate, or intensify the production of these harmful estrogen products, especially in embryos. These include pesticides, solvents, the manufacturing by-product dioxin, and the synthetic estrogen DES, which is fed to livestock in the United States.

The importance of Dr. Cavalieri and others' work, as described above, is that we have clearly identified a major cancer initiator, and we know how to stop its destructive actions on cells.

It is appalling to contrast these scientific findings with the conventional practice of prescribing estrogen replacement therapy (ERT) using estrogen alone to women without a uterus, or HRT using progestins instead of progesterone. Progestins are not progesterone and certainly do not provide the vital intracellular message that protects against breast cancer.

❖ WHAT YOUR ONCOLOGIST MAY NOT TELL YOU ABOUT TAMOXIFEN

A woman named Deborah wrote to Dr. Lee looking for reassurance that it would be safe for her to use progesterone cream. She had been diagnosed with breast cancer a year before, had been through chemotherapy and radiation, and was then put on tamoxifen. Her most recent tests were showing that she was free of cancer, but she had developed an "allergic" reaction to the tamoxifen, and her oncologist wanted to put her on a progestin instead. Deborah was well aware of the dangers of the progestins. Her doctor acknowledged the dangers but didn't know where else to turn to find a drug that would oppose or block estrogen, which stimulates breast cancers.

Deborah told her doctor about transdermal natural progesterone cream, but he wasn't aware that progestins are different from progesterone and was very uneasy about using a product that didn't fall into the category of a "standard of medical care."

Deborah decided she was on her own, and that's when she contacted Dr. Lee. He told her that if he were in her position he would definitely use progesterone cream. He also told her he personally knows many women who had breast cancer surgery, who thereafter used progesterone cream, and who are all cancer-free now, some of them as much as two decades later.

It's extremely scary for a woman who has stared down breast cancer, who has been through chemotherapy and radiation, and who knows she will spend the rest of her life wondering if it has come back, to try treatments that don't fall within the boundaries of conventional medicine.

A widely publicized recent study by the National Cancer Institute (NCI) showed that tamoxifen helps prevent breast cancer. Women who participated in the study were quoted in the media as saying that even though tamoxifen has serious side effects, the study will lead to better drugs to prevent breast cancer.

Deborah was told by her doctor that tamoxifen only increases the risk of uterine cancer by 1 percent. However, other researchers claim that the numbers are closer to 70 percent. Let's take a closer look at the real story behind tamoxifen.

Tamoxifen is a synthetic, nonsteroid, weakly acting estrogenic drug that effectively binds to estrogen receptors. The theory is that tamoxifen reduces one's breast cancer risk by blocking stronger estrogens such as human estrone and estradiol. Most doctors think of tamoxifen as an "antiestrogen." In the present NCI study, 13,000 women were given either tamoxifen or a placebo. Reportedly, 154 of the women receiving the placebo developed invasive breast cancer, while only 85 women on tamoxifen did. That is, for every 1000 women placed on tamoxifen, about 9 women (or about one woman in 100) would be spared the development of invasive breast cancer. The study had been planned to extend longer but was cut short, it is claimed, so those women on the placebo could switch to tamoxifen. This is in direct contrast to two European studies (Powles and Veronesi) that were smaller but of longer duration, which show no protective effect of tamoxifen.

Tamoxifen first appeared on the medical scene twenty-five years ago. After 5 years of use, it was found that the cancer-protective benefit waned. Moreover, numerous serious side effects of the drug emerged. It has been clearly established in both animal and human studies that tamoxifen quickly causes thickening of the uterus (considered a precursor to cancer) in virtually all test subjects. Tamoxifen is sufficiently estrogenic to cause endometrial (uterine) cancer and is listed by the World

Health Organization (WHO) as a cancer-causing drug. NCI director Richard D. Klausner also noted that, among the women taking tamoxifen, 33 developed uterine cancer compared with only 14 in the placebo group.

Other side effects include a tripling of the risk of potentially fatal blood clots in the lung and increased risk of stroke, blindness, and liver dysfunction. In fact, it has never been shown that tamoxifen reduced the mortality rate of women using it, regardless of its "protection" against breast cancer. All this has been known for twenty years. Clearly, tamoxifen will not solve the breast cancer problem.

The most valuable information to be gained from this study is that it makes it even more clear that breast cancer is due to long-term unopposed estrogen exposure (estrogen dominance) and that tamoxifen is not the answer to the problem. Short of castrating (removing the ovaries of) women to obliterate their estrogen production, what treatment is available to protect them from unopposed estrogen? Fortunately, the treatment is relatively simple and even wholesome, and it has to do, not surprisingly, with avoiding estrogen dominance and maintaining hormone balance as much as possible.

❧ THE EMOTIONAL SIDE OF BREAST CANCER

Breast cancer has been well studied, and out of all this research, a very clear breast cancer personality has emerged. She is the woman who can give to everyone else, but cannot, or is not allowed to, receive. She'll go to the grocery store to buy favorite foods for everyone in the family, but if you ask her what her own favorite foods are she may not even know. Dr. Hanley describes this as the shut-down of a woman's own nourishing and nurturing cycle, and the breasts are a symbol of nourishment. When the self-nourishing cycle is broken, the self-nourishing en-ergy becomes stuck in the breasts.

Dr. Hanley, who comes from a family with a high risk for breast cancer, teaches her women patients to do breast exams and finds that women who become familiar with their breasts can detect an abnormal lump very early on.

She also recommends doing a breast massage that is based on an old Taoist Chinese exercise that is part of a women's energy healing. This daily ritual massages the breasts in a circular motion, stimulating both the circu-lation and the lymph passages and glands, which are plentiful around the breast. It can be done every morn-ing in the shower.

Dr. Hanley teaches women that they don't have to be afraid to touch their breasts. When women have experi-enced a lot of fear of breast cancer or have had painful and tender breasts, she encourages them to say to their breasts as they massage them, "I'm taking care of you." A woman who massages her breasts regularly will have an intimate knowledge of their unique architecture and will become familiar with the changes that occur at different times through the menstrual cycle. Some women become fearful when their breasts become lumpier premenstrually. A woman who massages her breasts will be comfortable with those changes.

Dr. Hanley also believes that the massage literally clears away the herbicides, pesticides, and other dangerous chemicals that lodge in the fatty tissues of the breasts. A woman who is consciously taking care of her breasts feels more powerful because she is able to participate in her own protection, her prevention, and her early diagnosis of an unusual lump.

Dr. Hanley also encourages her patients not to wear underwire bras, or even tight bras, except for special occasions because they block the lymph glands underneath the breasts. Lymph glands play an important role in draining toxins from the breast.

Dr. Hanley also recommends a regular program of detoxification and cleansing for women who have a high risk of any type of cancer. This can include something as simple as eating a high-fiber vegetarian diet for a few days a month to a formalized cleansing program that utilizes special herbs and nutrients. (For details, see page 402.) The cleansing process rejuvenates the liver, which is responsible for clearing out excess hormones and their by-products.

Fresh, raw vegetable juices are also very cleansing and detoxifying, and they provide concentrated sources of enzymes and nutrients. Be sure to use organic produce to avoid getting a concentrated dose of pesticides. Use carrot and beet juice in small amounts because they are very high in sugar. There are many good books available on using fresh juices for healing. Some are listed in the Recommended Reading list at the back of the book.

❖ DR. LEE'S BASIC BREAST CANCER ❖ PREVENTION PROGRAM

If the following recommendations were followed by the majority of women, we would see the incidence of hormone-related cancers (and probably other cancers) plummet within a generation.

- Limit your consumption of sugar, refined carbohydrates (pasta, white bread, white rice), trans–fatty acids (hydrogenated oils, margarines, fried foods), and estrogen-rich foods such as feed-lot meat and cows' milk. Increase your consumption of foods with sulfated amino acids, such as beans, onions, and garlic.
- To prevent higher risk of cancer in our children, women (and men) contemplating pregnancy should avoid xenobiotics such as food containing pesticides and insecticide residue, and eat organically grown food. They should also avoid processed foods as much as possible because they contain harmful dyes and a potpourri of other chemicals with unknown effects. Also avoid all types of pesticides, herbicides, and fungicides, including household sprays, insecticide "bombs," and lawn and garden chemicals. This is also an

important step for prevention of breast cancer and prostate cancer in adults.

- Women must become aware that hormone imbalance starts progressively earlier in industrialized countries. Progesterone levels may become deficient by age twenty-five or thirty, and this deficiency affects about 50 percent of women by age thirty-five in the United States, thus creating estrogen dominance. When hormone-level testing or symptoms indicate estrogen dominance, progesterone should be supplemented.

- Foreign progesterone-like prescription compounds, such as those found in Provera and in birth control pills, should not be confused with real progesterone and should be avoided. Birth control pills play an important role in creating early hormone imbalances and should be avoided if at all possible.

- Even after menopause, estrogen (estrone) is still being created by body fat. Preventive low-dose progesterone supplementation (12–15 mg per day) can be used 24 to 25 days per month. Estrogen supplementation should only be used if indicated by vaginal dryness or thinning, night sweats, or unremitting hot flashes. The correct dose is the lowest dose that prevents these symptoms. Estriol is safer in regard to breast cancer than estrone or estradiol.

- Prescriptions for unopposed estrogen should be banned. No woman should ever be given estrogen without progesterone, even if she doesn't have a uterus or ovaries. Furthermore, there is no reason to believe that progestins such as Provera are as beneficial as real progesterone when it comes to preventing cancer. When estrogen supplementation is indicated, it should be preceded by progesterone supplementation, and the estrogen dosage should be kept as low as possible. Since progesterone restores normal estrogen receptor sensitivity, maintaining normal progesterone levels decreases the need for estrogen supplementation while at the same time preventing undesirable estrogen side effects.

- Progesterone replacement with a transdermal cream should be used prior to surgery by all patients having breast cancer surgery.

- Progesterone supplementation should be maintained for life with all breast cancer patients, before, during, and after surgery.

- All women with a family history of breast cancer should be closely monitored to avoid estrogen dominance.

✦ ENDOMETRIAL (UTERINE) CANCER AND HORMONES

Endometrial cancer is a relatively uncommon cancer and an even more rare cause of death. It is not among the five leading cancers in women of any age, nor is it among the ten leading cancer sites that include both men and women. In the United States it accounts for 2.6 deaths per 100,000 women, approximately one-tenth that of breast cancer and one-fifth that of cancer of the colon and rectum. Endometrial cancer is generally slow-growing and rarely metastasizes to distant sites in the body. The usual time in a woman's life when endometrial cancer develops is during the stage when she is estrogen dominant because progesterone levels have fallen premenopausally, due to anovulatory cycles, but estrogen levels remain normal.

Endometrial cancer is usually diagnosed by an exploratory surgery called dilation and curettage (D&C) or by endometrial biopsy in postmenopausal women with abnormal vaginal bleeding. Removing the uterus usually cures endometrial cancer.

The only known cause of endometrial cancer is unopposed estrogen. Estrogen stimulates endometrial hyperplasia (abnormal cell growth) and can lead eventually to endometrial cancer. Progesterone opposes this estrogen effect. This information has been a standard part of medical education for a generation but it seems to have been forgotten by doctors who prescribe HRT based on drug company advertising.

In the early 1970s, the widespread use of estrogen replacement therapy (ERT) resulted in an obvious increase of endometrial cancer: six to eight times greater occurrence in women using ERT than in women not using ERT. In 1976 this led to a change in hormone replacement therapy to include a progestin for postmenopausal women with an intact uterus. This is known now as HRT, or hormone replacement therapy.

In 1993 a comparison of 142 women who had endometrial cancer with 1,042 control subjects found that use of oral contraceptives, most of which contain progestin-like synthetic hormones, was partially protective against endometrial cancer. The use of unopposed estrogen without a progestin was an independent factor increasing the risk of endometrial cancer. In other words, even a synthetic, progesterone-like hormone, such as oral contraceptive progestins, conveys some protection against endometrial cancer as compared with estrogen alone.

Also in 1993 a group of researchers led by K. Boman reported in the journal *Cancer* that the proliferative activity of endometrial cancer cells fell, and the cells were well to moderately differentiated, when women's naturally occurring progesterone serum levels were high enough. At low progesterone levels, the cells were less differentiated and the proliferation rate was higher.

The 1995 study known as the PEPI (postmenopausal estrogen/progestin interventions) trial, in which 875 healthy postmenopausal women were randomly assigned to different treatment groups including placebo, unopposed estrogen, estrogen with progestin, and estrogen with oral progesterone and were followed for three years to evaluate the hormones' effect on potential heart risk factors. As an incidental observation, the PEPI study found equivalent protection against endometrial hyperplasia by both a progestin (medroxyprogesterone acetate, also known as Provera) and progesterone (oral micronized progesterone).

Two women (one in the unopposed estrogen group and one receiving placebo) developed localized endometrial cancer and were treated by hysterectomy. Twelve other women on unopposed estrogen were treated by hysterectomy because of atypia, adenomatous hyperplasia, fibroid tumor, pelvic mass, or abnormal vaginal bleeding, all estrogen-induced abnormalities. Thirty-four percent of the women on unopposed estrogen developed atypical hyperplasia. None of the women using either progesterone or the progestin along with estrogen supplementation developed hyperplasia, or required hysterectomy for any reason.

Dr. Lee has observed six patients who were diagnosed (by other physicians) as having endometrial cancer by D&C or biopsy while on ERT. After discontinuing estrogen and restoring normal progesterone levels by use of transdermal progesterone cream, repeat biopsies have found no cancer cells. These women have been followed for six to eighteen years now and have no sign of endometrial cancer. Because endometrial cancer is relatively slow-growing, most women should be able to safely try using progesterone before having a hysterectomy.

❧ MEN, HORMONES, AND CANCER

Just as the testicles are the male equivalent of the female ovaries, the prostate is the male equivalent of the female uterus; in both cases they originate from the same embryonic cells. It should not be surprising then that we see the same hormonal effects in both the prostate and the uterus. Dr. Lee, Dr. Hanley, and increasing numbers of other clinicians and researchers believe that it is excessive exposure to estrogen that is the primary cause of prostate enlargement and prostate cancer. Dozens of anecdotal reports of both reduction of enlarged prostates and reversal of prostate cancers through direct application of small amounts of progesterone cream appear to be preliminary evidence that progesterone may also play an important role in protecting the prostate gland in men. We hope that this theory is tested by research in the very near future.

❧ OVARIAN CANCER AND HORMONES

As we mentioned in chapter 7, ovarian cancer is particularly scary because by the time it's detectable, in 70 to 80 percent of women it has already spread to other parts of the body and thus has a high mortality rate. It accounts for nearly 20 percent of gynecologic cancers, and it ranks fifth in cancer fatalities in women. Most ovarian cancer occurs in menopausal women around the age of fifty.

The best way that your physician has of diagnosing ovarian cancer is by palpation (feeling the ovaries with the hands) during a pelvic exam. Younger women will frequently have enlarged or "functional" cysts on their ovaries, and most doctors will give the cysts six weeks to disappear—which they usually do—before doing exploratory surgery. Menopausal women in their fifties have smaller ovaries that normally aren't detectable with palpation, so the presence of a larger ovary in a menopausal woman can be cause for alarm.

Benign (noncancerous) ovarian cysts are very common in premenopausal women, and as the cysts go through the process of "resolving" or dissolving, they can create all manner of symptoms, including abdominal pain and bloating; sharp pains, and cramps; a feeling of indigestion; and, sometimes, irregular bleeding. Between erratic ovaries and an occasionally fussy uterus that cramps, most women become accustomed to sporadic aches and pains in that part of the body, so the symptoms of ovarian cancer may go unnoticed until it is affecting other parts of the pelvic cavity. Symptoms of excessive or deficient estrogen, progesterone, or androgens (male hormones) can also be symptoms of ovarian cancer, as the tumor may create an excess or deficiency of these hormones. These are symptoms that could easily be dismissed by a premenopausal woman whose hormones are fluctuating. In most cases, these types of symptoms are not cause for alarm until you are menopausal. If you are menopausal, you should see your doctor about them.

It has become clear that one of the causes of the increasing rate of ovarian cancer is the widespread use of fertility drugs that stimulate the ovaries to mature follicles.

The longer the drugs are used, the more the risk of ovarian cancer increases. One study found that using fertility drugs increased ovarian cancer risk three times, but in women who had never been pregnant the risk was increased 27-fold. Other studies have shown that women who are infertile and women who delay childbearing also have a higher risk of ovarian cancer, so a woman who uses fertility drugs may be significantly increasing an already elevated risk. Dr. Hanley is particularly concerned that the increasing use of fertility drugs by thousands of women, combined with the prevalence of estrogen dominance, may create an epidemic of ovarian cancer in the next few decades.

Your risk of ovarian cancer is also increased if you have a relative who has had it, if your consumption of dairy products is high, and if you use talcum powder. It is thought that the powder, which contains toxins such as heavy metals, migrates up the vagina, through the cervix, into the uterus and onto the ovaries.

The more full-term pregnancies a woman has had, the lower her statistical risk of ovarian cancer. Pregnancy is a time when the ovaries get a rest for nine months, and some researchers believe that the continuous ovulation of women who haven't had a full-term pregnancy increases the risk that a cancerous cyst will form. During pregnancy, progesterone levels are very high. As we've discussed, high progesterone levels provide protection against cancer.

A 1995 study by C. Rodriquez and associates published in the *American Journal of Epidemiology* showed that in 240,073 women studied, the relative risk of fatal ovarian cancer was 72 percent greater among those women who were given unopposed estrogen for six years or more. This study by Emory University School of Public Health and the American Cancer Society, which followed premenopausal and postmenopausal women for eight years, found that this risk was not modified by any of the other risk factors such as age at menarche, age of menopause, previous contraceptive use, tubal ligation, family history, body mass index, or education. The authors concluded that "long-term use of estrogen replacement therapy may increase the risk of fatal ovarian cancer."

This supports the hypothesis that estrogen dominance significantly increases the risk of fatal ovarian cancer. However, estrogen dominance is not limited merely to those women who are receiving unopposed estrogen. As you've learned from reading this book, premenopausal women are often estrogen dominant. If the comparison in the Rodriquez study had been made between ERT women and those who were not estrogen dominant for any reason, the risk ratio of the ERT group would have been considerably higher.

Part III

THE PREMENOPAUSE BALANCE PROGRAM

Practical Steps for Optimal Health

Chapter 13

❖

Restoring and Maintaining Balance

Janet was a very slim, fit, athletic, sports-oriented California-born-and-bred thirty-six-year-old whose life revolved around backpacking, skiing, mountain climbing, surfing, and river rafting. She and her husband worked for a large outdoor clothing and equipment company and were frequently sent off on trips to exotic locales to do photographic shoots for the company's mail order catalogue. Wherever they were, they always scheduled some type of outdoor adventure. They didn't have a lot of money, they didn't own a house, and their car was an old junker, but they felt incredibly lucky to be paid for doing what they loved best.

When Janet had her first appointment with Dr. Hanley, she tried to be casual and offhand about her symptoms, but Dr. Hanley could tell there were tears lurking underneath the healthy-looking tan and smile on her face. Janet was slim, muscular, and very restless, rubbing her hands together, shifting positions in the chair, running her fingers through her hair, and talking animatedly. She told Dr. Hanley that during their last trip to Peru she hadn't been able to keep up with the rest of her group on a four-day backpack trip into the high Andes mountains. She felt deeply fatigued, and got out of breath easily. Her periods, she said, were often irregular and only lasted two or three days with very little bleeding, and she was used to that, but now they had disappeared altogether. She found herself feeling constantly cold, as she described it, "freezing," even in warm weather, and she felt weepy and discouraged, which, she assured Dr. Hanley, was not like her. She wasn't sleeping very well, waking up many times during the night, and found herself craving junk food.

When Dr. Hanley told Janet she was suffering from premenopause syndrome, Janet was very quick to say, "Oh no, I'm not ready for that. I'm not anywhere near menopause!" Janet's reaction is a common and understandable response to hearing a diagnosis that includes "menopause" when you're only in your mid-thirties. Janet was not only young, she was young at heart and still had many travel plans, as well as plans to have children.

"We'd like to think of a better name for what's happening to you," Dr. Hanley told her, "but we haven't found it yet. But don't worry, I'm sure menopause itself isn't going to come around to you for many years. You have plenty of time to live out your dreams, including having babies!"

Janet's light or nonexistent menstruation is commonly found among women athletes. When the body is pushed very hard physically it decides that it is not a good environment for making babies, and shuts down the reproductive function. But it was clear that Janet's body wasn't functioning well in other areas. Her cold hands and feet combined with fatigue gave Dr. Hanley a good clue that Janet's thyroid wasn't in good working order, and her craving for junk food was a clue that her diet needed some adjusting. Her restlessness, anxiety, and insomnia, combined with feelings of discouragement and weepiness, were hallmarks of estrogen dominance, which made sense since Janet obviously was not ovulating and thus not making any progesterone in her ovaries, which would have balanced the effects of the estrogen. When Dr. Hanley questioned her about the foods she ate, Janet admitted that the staple of her diet, especially when traveling, was an assortment of the so-called nutrition bars and fruit and very little in the way of fresh vegetables, meat, or fish.

Although Janet's thyroid tests came out normal, Dr. Hanley suspected that the dominant estrogen in her body was blocking her thyroid function. So rather than giving her thyroid supplements right away, she asked her to use a progesterone cream to find out if balancing the estrogen brought back the thyroid function.

Dr. Hanley also asked Janet to keep a daily journal of how she felt physically and emotionally so that she could gauge her progress and do some detective work about what besides estrogen dominance might be causing her symptoms. Six weeks after her first visit Janet returned to Dr. Hanley and confided that through the journal writing she had come to realize that she was tired of traveling and wanted to settle down in her own home and have children. She also realized that she had become jealous of the young models in their early twenties who went on the photo shoots with them, whose effortless youth and energy made her feel old, and that she was dreading their next trip.

Once Janet became aware of these feelings she was able to talk with her husband about them, and she found to her surprise that he was supportive of less travel for both of them. She also learned that he was not lusting after the young models and in fact valued their relationship more than ever. He wasn't quite ready to start having children, but thought he would be once they had a home and were more settled and secure.

Over the course of a year, with a combination of diet changes, herbs and progesterone cream, Janet found that she was menstruating regularly again and had her energy and enthusiasm back. She told Dr. Hanley that writing in her journal and becoming clear about what she needed for herself had been an important part of the puzzle, without which she wouldn't have been able to fully heal.

Janet's story is a good example of how premenopause syndrome can have a multitude of causes, including physical and emotional stress. There is no cookbook of recipes for curing premenopause syndrome and bringing the body back into balance. It's up to each woman to work out what her symptoms are and track down what might be causing them. Janet's healing came in restoring balance to her life on every level—the core of creating a healthy lifestyle.

✦ BRINGING BALANCE INTO YOUR LIFE

Believe it or not, the prescription for maintaining balance for the vast majority of women is this: Learn how to take care of yourself instead of taking care of everyone else except yourself. This doesn't mean being selfish or self-centered. Far from it. But how can you take care of your loved ones if you're sick? How can you help others have a high quality of life if your own quality of life is low?

Learning how to take care of yourself usually boils down to learning how to pay attention to what you need to stay in balance, or, to put it another way, learning how to pay attention to what throws you out of balance, and being willing to change it. The concept of bringing balance into your life is a beautiful one that can be applied to everything you think, say, and do. It can be equally applied to the physical, emotional, mental, and spiritual aspects of your life. Just taking an inventory of what's in balance and what's out of balance in your life is a remarkably eye-opening and healing process. You'd be amazed at how quickly life changes when you strive to bring the details of it into balance.

Sometimes we need help identifying which parts of ourselves are out of balance. Janet sensed that her life wasn't satisfying, but she couldn't quite figure out why.

On the surface she had everything she could wish for. The simple awareness that she was neglecting an important part of herself, and her willingness to change, opened up a whole new life for her. Greater awareness can come in the form of a spiritual teacher, a book, a journal, a creative hobby, a friend or relative, a member of the clergy, or a therapist. Sometimes it just takes a vacation to give us perspective on our lives.

One way to help bring your life into balance is to identify the areas where you're at an extreme in your life and then to take small, simple steps to begin to bring that part of your life back to center. For example, for Janet, just the realization that she wanted to "nest" more was healing in and of itself and had the happy side effect of improving her relationship with her husband. For Marie, the driven, zooming career woman described in chapter 1, simply walking through the hallways at work rather than running was a small step in the right direction of slowing down the pace of her life.

If you know that coffee is upsetting your stomach but you can't seem to quit the habit, start with a small step of drinking what is now called a "half-caff" coffee, which is half decaffeinated. If it's difficult for you not to be compulsive about keeping the house clean, and you tend to stay up past midnight vacuuming, begin with one room and let the dust bunnies collect under a piece of furniture there. On the other hand, if your house is so cluttered there's hardly space to walk between the piles, begin cleaning one small corner of one room. If you're a perfectionist about putting on a meal for your family every night, try using paper plates one or two nights a week. If you can't seem to get anything but fast food or TV dinners on the table, start with cooking a quick, simple dinner rather than a gourmet meal that involves hours of preparation. If you're the queen of incompletions and can never seem to finish anything you start, make a list and then begin by finishing one small task and crossing it off. If you make a goal of completing everything in a week, you're only setting yourself up for failure.

As you bring your life into balance, going to extremes to do it will just throw you into another state of imbalance. Be gentle with yourself. If there's no way you're ever going to let a dust bunny be born under your couch, find another area of your life to ease up on.

Most women in the midcycle of life are trying to do too much, and that in and of itself is a setup for a hormonal imbalance. But there are some strategies for staying more centered that can apply to most premenopausal women. Here's a thumbnail sketch that can get you started with your own personal list.

- Don't turn on the TV every night.
- Switch from coffee to tea (green tea is best).
- Limit alcohol consumption to one drink with dinner—eliminate it if it makes you tired or sleepy.
- Listen to soothing music or books on tape in the car. Or, if you have kids, talk to them. Reserve the car phone for emergencies. Leave early and drive the speed limit.

- Learn to say no when you're about to add another responsibility to your life that you can't handle.
- Indulge in some form of meditation or meditative exercise such as chi gong or yoga and have some type of spiritual practice or higher purpose in your life. This gives you a "place" inside of yourself to go when things get tough outside.
- If you have children, remember to keep track of your own needs as well as theirs, and find ways to meet your needs even if it means not meeting their needs perfectly.
- If there are two working adults in the house, split housework and cooking fairly. Forget about being superwoman.
- Don't have sex with your partner unless you really want to, and then speak up if something about it is bothering you.
- Tell your partner if something is bothering you. Don't let small irritations build up into anger.
- Get some type of exercise every day. That doesn't have to mean a trip to the gym for a killer ninety minutes of aerobics. It can mean a walk after dinner, a bike ride with the kids, or some time in the garden. The point is to move your body.
- Eat whole, natural foods (preferably organic), drink plenty of clean water, and take a good multivitamin.
- Avoid prescription drugs, surgery, and hospitals whenever possible. Find a doctor or other health care professional who shares your values about health and healing.

- On the financial front, keep spending within reasonable limits.
- Leave an abusive work or home situation if you can't change it. This includes mental, emotional, and physical abuse. If you are an abuser, get counseling.
- If you're lonely, find someplace to volunteer where you will be helping others.
- Get plenty of sleep.
- Ask for help when you need it and express gratitude when you get it.
- Take time to do things that make you laugh.
- Be kind to yourself, forgive yourself, refrain from judging yourself harshly. Give yourself a break.
- Avoid being strict or righteous about anything.
- Keep in touch with friends and family.
- Recognize, accept, and acknowledge out-of-balance emotions, but at the same time, take a dispassionate view of them. They aren't to be ignored, but they aren't to be worshipped either.

❧ YOUR OWN PERSONAL JUGGLING ACT

As your hormones begin to go through their premenopausal fluctuations you'll be able to maintain balance more effectively if you're attuned to your body, your emotions, and your mind. Each aspect of yourself will give you valuable clues about what's out of balance and then you have a choice, based on your own personal preferences, of how to restore balance.

For example, if you notice that your hands and feet

are cold, that could be a clue that your thyroid is under-performing. The cause could be a side effect of estrogen dominance blocking thyroid function, or it could be a true thyroid deficiency. You could stimulate your thyroid and restore balance by eating an iodine-containing sea vegetable such as nori or kombu. You could go to your health food store and get a supplement designed to boost thyroid function with glandular thyroid and amino acids. Or you could go to your doctor and have your thyroid function tested.

If you're retaining water or your face is flushed, there's a good chance that you are estrogen dominant. If you are also constipated it may be that you're not eating enough fiber and your liver is having trouble excreting the estrogen normally handled by fiber. In that case you could do something as simple as having a bran muffin or as involved as having your hormone levels tested.

If you're dragging yourself out of bed in the morning, your adrenal function may not be up to par. You have a range of options to choose from to bring your adrenals back into balance that range from staying in bed for another hour (or the day) and resting, which will help a lot, drinking some licorice or ginseng tea, taking some DHEA or hydrocortisone, or all of the above.

By the time you finish reading this book, you will have enough clues as to what's out of balance so that most of the time you can take corrective action. But remember, it's rarely going to be a matter of just tweaking your thyroid, reducing your estrogen, or supporting your adrenals. Remember the hormonal symphony? Supporting individual symptoms will help, but it's the whole orchestra playing in unison that creates harmony. You'll generally need to take action on more than one level. What else is going on in your life? Are you getting enough sleep? Are you eating fresh vegetables? Have you taken a walk lately? Did you sit in traffic and breathe car exhaust on the way home from a stressful day at work? If you fail to address the underlying causes, you may get the violin section tuned up but the horns will have fallen asleep.

How you choose to bring harmony to your own hormonal symphony is a purely individual matter. Some women become adept at juggling nutritional and hormonal supplements, while others look to foods such as soy and fresh vegetable juices, and still others depend on an hour a day at the gym. It could be that doing some yoga, taking a bubble bath, or getting a good laugh watching your favorite sitcom is what you need to restore balance.

❖ THE LISTENING AND DEEPENING PROCESS

Symptoms are your body's way of telling you that something is out of balance. If you listen well and respond with care, you will be rewarded with better health and you'll spend less time, energy, and money on maintaining balance. On the other hand, not stopping to heed your body's early warnings can lead to more serious problems. Ignoring mild heartburn can eventually lead to an ulcer.

Ignoring fatigue can lead to exhaustion. Ignoring mild pain in a joint can lead to chronic inflammation. It's relatively easy to treat the underlying causes of mild heartburn, fatigue, or pain, and it's a major undertaking to treat the more serious consequences that can result when you ignore those symptoms. The same applies to hormone balance.

If you're used to ignoring your body, one of the best ways to begin learning to listen to it is to keep a daily journal where you list anything you've noticed during the day, ranging from feeling weepy to a cramp in your little toe to dry skin to high energy or clear thinking. Eventually you'll begin to notice patterns of cause and effect and you'll be able to work with the cause instead of the effect. That's called prevention.

This is not to suggest that you should necessarily avoid working with a health care professional. Unless you're a unique woman, you can't see or hear or feel cervical cancer happening, so it's a good idea to have a pap smear every few years (more often if you've been taking oral contraceptives). You can't detect osteoporosis when it begins at thirty-five, so it pays to get a bone density test in your mid-thirties so that you have a baseline to work with. If you're having irregular bleeding that your efforts don't help after a few months, then it's important to see a physician to rule out endometrial cancer.

While you are premenopausal, for ten or even twenty years, your body is not always going to behave in a predictable way. It's not going to fall into any set parameters or fixed numbers that can be measured or reliably be called normal, average, or standard. You need to become your own best expert on what's right and normal and best for you. As you age and become more sensitive to environmental toxins, you're more likely to notice toxic effects. A young woman may be able to sit in traffic with the car windows open or douse the house with a can of ant spray and not notice any effects. An older woman may notice sinus congestion, dry eyes, or swelling in the face and hands.

Around the age of thirty-five, you are entering a life cycle where you have lived long enough that you have formed your own ideas. You have taken ideas and experiences from your parents, friends, lovers, schools, and religious institutions and woven them into a fabric of your psyche that is the beginning of wisdom and understanding. Your body is becoming more sensitive to environmental, dietary, and emotional influences, and your mind and emotions are more sensitive to your own—and others'—inner and outer dynamics.

The more you embrace this wonderful transformation, and honor and respect yourself now, the smoother the ride you'll have in the long run. As you get closer to menopause you'll be amazed at your growing powers of perception in almost all facets of your life. These are qualities that make a mature woman so inherently valuable to her family and her community.

Dr. Hanley worked with a woman named Claudia who had been diagnosed by her physician as having gone into early menopause at the age of thirty-four. She was having hot flashes and night sweats, her hormone levels were fluctuating all over the place, and an ultrasound showed that she had some ovarian cysts.

At their first meeting, Dr. Hanley asked her if there had been anything severely traumatic that had gone on in her life in the past few years, and Claudia went on to tell Dr. Hanley a tragic story. Her first child was born with a rare disease that doomed him to a very difficult life. When she got pregnant again, against her better judgment, she was told that her second child could never have the disease because the first one had been a genetic mutation. But just a few weeks later they found out that her husband had the disease, and then genetic testing showed that the second child had it too, so she had an abortion. Soon after the abortion she went into menopause.

Claudia had asked the physician treating her at the time if the trauma and shocks of the past few years could have created her premature menopause, and her physician had told her it had nothing to do with it, that she was just one of those women who goes into early menopause. He recommended that her ovaries be removed because of the ovarian cysts and that she then take synthetic hormones. Claudia knew in her heart that her physician wasn't right, and that's when she made an appointment to see Dr. Hanley.

Dr. Hanley assured Claudia that the tragedies in her life had almost certainly caused her to go into premature menopause. After six months of working with her emotional scars and using natural hormones and herbs to support her body, her symptoms gradually went away and she began having menstrual cycles again. A follow-up ultrasound showed that her ovarian cysts had disappeared.

Had Claudia just gone along with what her doctor recommended, against her inner knowing, she would have been plunged into premature menopause for real, as well as a whole new set of problems caused by taking synthetic hormones that her body didn't want or need at the time. What Claudia needed most was emotional nourishment and gentle support for her exhausted body.

We should never underestimate the power of our emotional lives to affect our bodies, or the inherent ability we have to understand ourselves and what we need, to bring ourselves into balance.

Chapter 14

❧

How Nutrition Affects Your Hormone Balance

Although natural progesterone can have wonderfully curative effects on the symptoms of premenopause syndrome, it works best when you eat wholesome foods, pay attention to possible food allergies, and take nutritional supplements. The rewards of eating a nutritious diet are more than worth the sacrifices. You'll decrease your risk of future heart disease, cancer, diabetes, osteoporosis, and arthritis. If your diet has consisted largely of high-calorie, nutrition-free foods such as candy bars and cookies, your energy and moods will improve dramatically. If you suffer from indigestion, gas, bloating, and constipation, you'll be happy to know that eliminating food allergens and good nutrition are nearly always a cure. You'll catch fewer colds and flus because your immunity will improve, it will be easier to drop excess fat, and your skin will clear up. In some cases, a well-designed, individualized diet, supplement, and exercise program is all that's needed to restore balance during the premenopause years and beyond. Depending on your exposure to xenohormones, you may well find that you don't need to use natural progesterone.

What are these magical foods you're supposed to be eating? Which of the endless diets touted this month is the one to follow? Which of the hundreds of supplements found on health food store shelves should you be taking? There's no one answer for everybody, but this chapter gives you enough guidelines to begin to create your own personal hormone balance program.

When Dr. Hanley sees a premenopausal woman for the first appointment, they have an in-depth discussion about diet. Some women are coming from a lifetime of hardly thinking about what foods they put in their mouths, except for those times they've tried to lose weight. The more ambitious have gone to the bookstore for the latest best-selling diet books. Some say they've tried the high-carbohydrate, low-fat diets and felt worse than ever, while others say they feel great on such a diet but can't seem to stick to it. Still others swear by the popular diet books that promote balanced intake of fat, protein, and carbohydrates, while some feel them to be too regimented, unpalatable, or hard to follow. There's a lot of frustration around food for most women, and this is especially true of premenopausal women who are starting to gain some serious weight for the first time in their lives and can't seem to do anything to stop it.

Your first assignment is to stop worrying so much about the weight gain. This is not in any way an encouragement to become obese but rather an entreaty to let go of the starving model ideal. To the extent that you accept your womanly body you will be giving that gift of acceptance to the next generation of women as well! Mother Nature designed women so that they would put on a little bit of weight premenopausally. It will get you through menopause more gracefully and protect you from osteoporosis and strokes. If you don't allow the weight gain to become obesity, the latest research shows that you won't be at a higher risk for heart attacks and cancer, especially if you keep your hormones balanced. You can assume that you are obese if your weight is interfering with your ability to move around physically or if it is causing weight-related problems such as diabetes, arthritis, and difficulty breathing.

In spite of the charts and graphs and studies put out by everyone from the American Heart Association to the federal government, *there is no one diet that is right for everyone.* Nobody can hand you a piece of paper or a book that tells you exactly what you need to eat unless they have collected a lot of data first. Anyone who has done the work of figuring out their ideal foods and supplements can tell you that it's a process that takes some time, attention, and tracking. It takes trying new things. It means getting rid of the processed foods you depend on for comfort and replacing them with real, nourishing, substantial whole foods. It also means paying close attention to how your body responds to different foods and eliminating those that are having adverse effects on your health. No one can do this for you. The good news is that it can be a fun piece of detective work with great rewards.

You'll need to experiment to find out what foods are best for you and which nutrients you need more or less of. Vitamin C is highly recommended by just about every educated, knowledgeable health expert, yet some people react badly to it. (The recent study showing that vitamin C caused DNA damage is extremely inconclusive and is counterbalanced by hundreds of studies clearly showing its benefits, so please don't stop taking your vitamin C.) Complex carbohydrates such as brown rice and whole-grain wheat have a long list of health benefits, but some people just can't eat them without suffering from gas and indigestion. You need to find out what's best for *you*.

For years we've been told that a high-carbohydrate, low-fat diet was the best thing for us, and now the pendulum of popular opinion is swinging back toward diets high in protein and fat with very little carbohydrate. Neither works very well for the average person.

On a high-carbohydrate, low-fat diet, most people find they're always hungry and turn to refined carbs such as candy and baked goods to satisfy their cravings. They often end up overweight and malnourished. For most women, diets low in fat and protein lead to frequent dips in blood sugars. When we learn to build fires, we're taught that we need to start with tiny little twigs. But you don't light the fire until you have bigger branches to keep it going. If you live on carbohydrates, you are living on twigs. You light the twigs and try to venture out to find bigger sticks to keep it going, but the fire keeps going out and you constantly have to return to relight it.

At the other end of the spectrum is the high-protein, and high-fat diet, which makes most people feel sluggish and a little ill. Part of the reason people lose weight on these diets is because the body has no other fuel to burn but fat and protein, which don't supply the fuel for bursts of energy. It takes a lot of work for the body to maintain itself without healthy carbohydrates. A diet of nothing but meat, seafood, eggs, high-fat dairy products, and occasional vegetables can acidify the body. Minerals are pulled from bones to buffer extra acid. It's like trying to start your fire with nothing but big logs. Without the carbos as kindling, it's very hard to get the fire going.

✤ THE BUILDING BLOCKS OF GOOD NUTRITION

There aren't any foods that are necessarily good for everybody. Each type of food—vegetables, fruits, grains, nuts and seeds, legumes, meat, poultry, and seafood—comes with its own set of advantages and drawbacks, and the only way you'll find out which it is for you is to experiment. Much of this chapter is devoted to giving you guidelines for experimentation.

The only category of food that is clearly good for

pretty much everyone is fresh, organic vegetables and fruits. But individual tolerance for the type of fruit or vegetable varies widely. For example, some people are allergic to the nightshade vegetables, which includes potatoes, tomatoes, peppers, and eggplants. Other don't do well with the cruciferous vegetables such as cabbage, broccoli, and cauliflower. Even with a vegetable family you may be able to tolerate some members but not others. For example, some people have a hard time digesting onions but do fine with garlic.

A wide variation exists in the ability to tolerate fruits. Grapes have a very high sugar content, so if your blood sugar tends to fluctuate easily, this may not be the fruit for you. Although apples are a popular fruit, they do give some people stomach cramps. Citrus fruits are high on the list of foods that cause allergies, but pears are almost universally tolerated.

Fresh fish and fresh, hormone-free meats (not cured or processed meats) are widely tolerated, but many people these days have ethical and moral concerns about eating meat. If you do eat meat and you're one of those people who digests meat well, you can relax in knowing that all nonprocessed, organic meat is good for you in moderation. It's not the beef, pork, or lamb per se that contributes to heart disease; it's including enormous quantities of fatty meat in your diet that will throw you off balance.

Beans or legumes such as soybeans provide a good source of fiber, protein, and other nutrients, but they can also be a source of painful gas and bloating. We'll give you more details on soy in particular later in the chapter.

Grains are also a mixed blessing. Whole grains offer a rich and valuable mix of nutrients, fiber and carbohydrates. But wheat in particular and gluten-containing grains in general are near the top of the list of allergy-containing foods. And as anyone who has tried to eliminate wheat from their diet can tell you, it's in so many things that it is very difficult to avoid.

Dairy products are very rich in nutrients, but, again, they come with their own set of potential problems and are a very common allergen. The milk pasteurization process, which is designed to kill harmful organisms, also kills all the enzymes and beneficial bacteria present that you need in order to digest milk properly. Milk also has a poor calcium to magnesium ratio which makes it a poor source of calcium for building bones.

Nuts and seeds are wonderfully nutritious foods, packed with nutrients and good oils. But they go rancid easily and if they're roasted at high heat, salted, and covered with peanut oil, much of their value will be lost. (Rancid oils smell bad. Fresh oils smell fresh.) Your best bet is to buy raw nuts and seeds and either eat them raw or roast them yourself for no more than ten minutes (on a cookie sheet at 350 degrees Fahrenheit). Be sure to store them in an airtight container, out of the sun, and eat them within a week or two.

Nuts and seeds also contain hundreds and maybe thousands of phytochemicals (plant compounds), many that we don't even know about yet, that can have a wide variety of effects on the body. The biggest nut allergen is peanuts, which are also often rancid. Choose your peanut butter and roasted peanuts with care, avoiding hydrogenated oils and sugar. Make sure it's fresh when you buy it (it should be dated), keep it in the refrigerator, and throw it away if it smells rancid.

Begin to think of food as a medicine that has a specific effect on your body and mood, because that's exactly what it is. What you eat can affect everything from your mental alertness to your physical strength and, you guessed it, your hormone balance. If you eat too little cholesterol, your body won't have the building blocks it needs to manufacture your ovarian and adrenal hormones (75 percent of your cholesterol is made from carbohydrates, but the remaining 25 percent comes from fats and oils). Eating a lot of sugar will cause ups and downs in your adrenaline and cortisol levels that will throw the rest of your hormones out of balance and make you feel anxious. When blood sugar is down you'll feel weak, irritable, and mentally slow. Eating plenty of fiber will help your colon sweep excess estrogen and other toxins out of the body. Too little fiber and they will be recycled back into the liver.

Tracking your response to a particular food will be easier if you keep a journal of what you eat and how you're feeling. As you read through the guidelines in the rest of this chapter, you'll gain confidence in your ability to discover the foods that are best for you.

Dr. Hanley's history is typical of the baby-boomer woman. She was born to a mother who smoked, she was bottle-fed with formula, and was raised on a steady diet of TV dinners and cows' milk. She was constantly ill and taking antibiotics for the first fifteen years of her life. When she was seventeen, she became a vegetarian with the help of a friend. A vegetarian diet got her free of many foods that were deleterious to her body and were causing her to be ill and exhausted. The cleansing effects of her new diet, which encouraged her body to engage its own natural detoxification processes, gave Dr. Hanley a new lease on life. However, as she approached midlife she found that she was out of balance again, dealing with persistent fatigue and illness. Adding meat and healthful fats back into her diet to bring it into better balance, and using supplements to fill the gaps, she became her present slimmer, healthier, more energetic self. Not that she's resting on her laurels—she knows that as her body undergoes the changes of perimenopause and menopause, she too will have to make adjustments here and there.

❖ THINK OF PROCESSED FOODS AS THE ENEMY

If the words *low fat* or *nonfat* are printed on a package, it must be healthful, right? It would be better if those words made you run the other way. Low-fat diets have led us *not* to eat more vegetables, fruits, and whole grains but rather to eat more refined carbohydrates, which means grains with all the nutrients stripped out of them and hydrogenated oils added. Low-fat and nonfat packaged chips, pretzels, breads, and pastries are part of most health-conscious American's larder, but they're bad food in disguise. Most often, low fat means high salt or high sugar, which is just trading one problem for another. Processed and packaged foods have very little that resembles nutrition left in them, and a lot added back in that is harmful to your health. The single best thing you can do for your health, your longevity, and your hormone balance is to learn to eat real, whole foods.

It wasn't too many generations ago that we had primarily whole, fresh foods on the dinner table because there weren't many other choices. Before the advent of refrigerators, freezers, and processed foods, a typical serving at dinner contained a modest portion of protein such as meat, poultry, or fish; a grain such as rice, potato, or whole grain bread; and a vegetable such as carrots, green beans, or broccoli. This is a wonderfully balanced meal of whole foods. It's relatively simple to prepare and balanced nutritionally for most people. We got off track when we started eating huge portions of protein; canned vegetables (if any); and huge portions of refined carbohydrates such as pasta, white rice, and white bread. Today we're lucky to have year-round access to a wide variety of fresh vegetables and fruits.

Regardless of your ethnic and cultural (and therefore dietary) heritage, if you go back far enough to the "native" diet that your ancestors ate, you'll find that it contains a balanced variety of whole foods.

❧ KICKING THE REFINED CARBOHYDRATE AND SUGAR HABIT

Refined carbohydrates (pasta, white bread, white rice, baked goods, chips, for example) are loaded with calories, but it's hard to consider them nutrition. They are calorically dense and low in the nutrients your body needs to feel satisfied, and they cause insulin secretion to be chronically high. Insulin is a fat-storage hormone, and the more of it there is in your bloodstream, the more of the calories you take in will be stored as fat. When you eat a meal high in refined carbohydrates, like a white-flour bagel with low-fat margarine and sugary jam, the lack of fiber, protein, and fat (all of which slow digestion and absorption) causes it to be digested rapidly. Once it hits the bloodstream and blood sugar levels spike, the pancreas has an alarm reaction, secreting enough insulin to pull all that sugar out of the blood. Remember, your pancreas is calibrated to respond to real food, not processed foods. Some of the glucose made from these foods passes into the cells throughout the body, and any extra is stored as glycogen (the storage form of glucose) or as fat. Then your blood sugar is low and you feel hungry again.

Processed sugar is an immunosuppressant and is terribly unbalancing, even more so than processed foods made from white flour. Its extremely intense sweet taste isn't found anywhere in the natural world, and for most people it has an addictive quality. Even the sweetest fruits, such as grapes, aren't as potent as processed sugar.

Let's face it, sugar is a drug. It's a white, powdered, crystalline substance that makes you want more and makes you cranky when you don't get it. Many women who have tried to cut their fat consumption way down have turned to treats loaded with sugar for their food fixes. There are no nutrients in sugar or other highly processed foods, and because your body needs nutrients to digest and assimilate what you eat, you end up drawing on your precious nutrient stores. Consumption of processed sugar is linked to heart disease just as strongly as overconsumption of fat. Even in small amounts, far below what the average American takes in every day, sugar impairs the functioning of the immune system.

When you eat a sugary snack like low-fat cookies or cake, frozen yogurt, or candy, that blood sugar spike and insulin overresponse sends your whole neuroendocrine system into emergency mode. Your adrenal glands pump out adrenaline to try to pick you back up after your blood sugar soars and dips precipitously down. It's truly a vicious cycle.

Both Dr. Lee and Dr. Hanley have repeatedly seen nutrient-poor junk foods cause severe behavioral and emotional problems in their patients. For many years Dr. Lee had treated a family that was very conscientious about the foods they ate. Their daughter Cindy went off to college on a scholarship and six months later Mom was calling Dr. Lee, asking for a referral to a psychiatrist because Cindy was sleepwalking, depressed, and getting low grades for the first time in her life.

Dr. Lee suggested that over spring break he talk to

Cindy. The first thing he asked her about is what she had been eating, and the answer was pasta, French fries, white bread, and ice cream. She was used to eating whole grains, and lots of fresh, organic vegetables and fruits, and suddenly she was immersed in junk food and sugar. Combined with the stress of being away from her family for the first time, it's no wonder things weren't going well!

She completely recovered while she was home for vacation, and when Cindy went back to college she found ways to bring her diet closer to what she had been eating at home and never had a recurrence of her problems.

People who have existed on processed foods from a young age tend to have a lot of resistance to giving them up for whole foods. In some cases, it's an issue of convenience. The preparation of meals from whole foods at home is more time-consuming (and less expensive) than tearing open a package or tossing a cardboard box into the microwave. You don't have to be a gourmet cook to eat whole foods. There are dozens of cookbooks, cooking classes, shows on TV, and magazine articles about quick, easy ways to cook whole foods. If you haven't been eating whole foods it will take some effort, but it's well worth it regardless of what else is going on in your life.

It can be very difficult to get kids who have been raised (so far) on processed foods to kick the habit. Why wouldn't they opt for a quick calorie fix and the taste of sugar if they can get it? One mother we know gets her kids to eat vegetables by putting out a plate of lightly salted carrot, celery, cucumber, zucchini, red pepper, and other vegetable sticks in the half hour before dinner when hunger pangs were setting in. Regardless of where the kids are—in front of the TV, studying, or outside playing basketball—the plate is always clean by the time dinner rolls around. On the other hand, the same plate of vegetables put on the dinner table wouldn't be touched. It only takes a few minutes to make a plate full of carrot and celery sticks, and if you get organic vegetables you won't even have to peel the carrots.

Some people are ferociously addicted to certain processed foods. We become addicted to refined carbohydrates because of that quick pick-me-up that turns into a blood sugar crash and a craving for more refined carbohydrates. Ironically, those are the foods that many women eat for comfort. Try to find comforts that don't involve large quantities of refined carbohydrates. Meditating, journal writing, exercising, or talking things over with a loved one are a few options to explore. It only takes a few days for the carbo cravings to die down. Dr. Hanley recommends that her patients who are kicking the carbo habit take 200 mcg daily of the trace mineral chromium picolinate to help stabilize blood sugar.

To kick your refined carbohydrate habit, gradually replace products made with white flour with whole grains like brown rice, amaranth, millet, quinoa, and bulgur. Buy whole-grain (not just whole wheat) or sprouted-grain breads (you'll need to read the labels carefully at first to find the healthful brands). Experiment with dried beans. If you soak them overnight and discard the soaking water before you cook them, they shouldn't cause gas.

Soy foods are big news right now, and there's a lot of promising research attesting to the phytoestrogens and other compounds they contain. All soy foods are not created equal, however, and that topic will be covered in more detail shortly.

Raw vegetables in a salad, lightly steamed vegetables (try the leafy green varieties like collards, kale, and spinach), baked root vegetables (beets, potatoes, yams, carrots, and turnips), and fruit to feed your sweet tooth are all nutrient-dense and naturally low in fat. The fats in whole foods are the ones our bodies need to build cell membranes, make cholesterol, and perform myriad other jobs. Even vegetables contain small amounts of fats—not enough to make you fatter but enough to nourish the cells that need these essential fatty acids to function. We have created a need for supplements such as flax seed oil, evening primrose oil, and borage oil because we are so deficient in the essential fatty acids found in whole grains, nuts, seeds, and fresh fruits and vegetables. Both eating foods stripped of their nutrients and eating hydrogenated oils have contributed to this deficiency. It's much healthier to get the essential fatty acids from whole foods than to take them in huge quantities as supplements that may or may not be rancid.

Cold-water fish that live far enough out at sea to avoid contamination by polluted shore or inland waters, are important sources of essential fats and other nutrients. Salmon, herring, mackerel, sardines, and cod are best. Albacore tuna is good too, but keep your consumption down to once a week since it can be contaminated with mercury. If you say "yuck" at the thought of fish, experiment until you find a type you like and a way to prepare it that makes it palatable. Most people like broiled salmon with lemon juice, and what could be more simple?

Suddenly switching to a whole-foods diet might cause some problems in your digestive tract, so make sure you do it gradually. You may want to invest in a good juicer as you start the shift. Fresh fruit and vegetable juices are excellent sources of concentrated nutrients for women short on time and energy. The enzymes contained in raw foods that help you digest them are intact when you make juice fresh and drink it right away. Don't overdo it, though—juices such as carrot juice, beet juice, and fruit juice can be a concentrated source of sugar as well, and they don't contain the important fiber you need for good digestion, detoxification, and clean bowels.

❧ NATURAL FATS AND OILS ARE GOOD FOR YOU

Don't believe the bad press fats are getting these days. The truth is that you need fat, including cholesterol-containing fat, in your diet. A very low-fat diet sends your body into an emergency response. The wisdom of the body perceives a famine and shuts down the ovaries, because if there isn't enough food for you, there's little chance of there being enough to maintain a pregnancy to term and produce a healthy infant. Anovulatory cycles set the stage for estrogen dominance. It is important, however, that you choose which kinds of fats you eat with care.

You need fat in your diet to build and maintain many aspects of your physiology, including cell membranes, cholesterol, and hormones. An imbalance of fats sets up an inflammatory situation in your body.

Prostaglandins are special kinds of hormones produced throughout the body. They maintain a variety of processes, including blood pressure and inflammation. Prostaglandin manufacture is largely driven by the fats and oils we eat. An excess of some types of prostaglandins causes hormone imbalance. The balance of "bad" hydrogenated and oxidized (rancid) polyunsaturated fats with "good" fats such as those found in fish, fresh vegetables and fruits, and olive oil dictates which prostaglandins are made. An imbalance means too many of the kind of prostaglandins that—in excess—cause inflammation, water retention, blood vessel constriction, and PMS.

Adequate and balanced intake of essential fatty acids (EFAs) can help keep your skin clear, your periods regular, and cramping to a minimum. Attention span and mood are improved with the right kind of fats in the diet. If you like to keep track of your fat and calorie intake, it's ideal for many women to keep total fat intake at 25 to 30 percent of total calories, no matter which fats you're eating. This is a very general guideline. For some women it may be 20 percent, and for others it may be 40 percent.

Rancid and partially hydrogenated oils comprise a significant portion of the fat intake of people in industrialized countries. Unstable or unsaturated oils such as corn, safflower, sunflower, peanut, and other nut and seed oils easily become oxidized. Much as a cut apple turns brown or a piece of metal rusts, these fat molecules become oxidized. Unstable polyunsaturated oils are readily transformed by the effects of heat and oxygen into harmful carriers of free radicals. Although a certain amount of free-radical production and oxidation is important to bodily processes, in excess they quickly damage proteins, cell membranes, and even DNA. Almost nobody in Western, industrialized countries is suffering from too little oxidation. Antioxidant nutrients such as vitamins C and E, the minerals zinc and selenium, and glutathione, some of which are found in foods and others of which are made in our bodies, protect our cells from free radicals by binding with and neutralizing them.

A hydrogenated oil is a liquid vegetable oil that's bombarded with hydrogen molecules to make it more solid and thus protect it from oxidation and rancidity. These unnatural oils are used in virtually all processed foods to make everything from margarines to baked goods to chips to frozen desserts. They have been very clearly and definitively linked to increased risk of artery disease. It seems that hydrogenated fats directly damage the delicate linings of blood vessels. They also throw off your hormone balance by blocking the actions of "good" EFAs. You'll most likely have fewer cramps and less PMS once you eliminate hydrogenated oils from your diet.

A recent Swedish study headed by Dr. Alicja Wolk and published in the *Archives of Internal Medicine*, analyzed more than 61,000 women between the ages of 40 and 70. Wolk and her colleagues found that while total fat intake was not related to breast cancer, the polyunsaturated fats found in vegetable oils increased the risk of cancer and the monounsaturated fats such as olive oil decreased the risk of cancer. As relatively little as 5 g unsaturated fat per day increased breast cancer risk by 69 percent. Saturated fats were not associated with an increase in breast cancer.

Saturated fats like butter, coconut oil, and lard are solid at room temperature, are very stable and are not susceptible to oxidation. You can leave them sitting out and not worry that they'll spoil, and you can heat them up without creating free radicals. Unrefined coconut oil and butter are best for baking. They won't oxidize when they're heated, and they have the best "mouth feel" of any fats in baked goods and candy. And no, eating saturated fats will *not* give you a heart attack unless you eat them in excess. Having a pat of butter on your toast in the morning is not going to kill you and will probably help your hormone balance. But stick to one piece of toast and eat some protein and fruit with it to create a balanced meal. Eating fatty red meat every day would create an excess of saturated fat.

Olive oil is a monounsaturated fat, meaning that it's liquid but is almost as stable as a saturated fat. Cultures that consume most of their fat as olive oil have lower incidences of heart disease and breast cancer. Always use olive oil before an unsaturated vegetable oil. Look for dark green extra-virgin olive oils. They're a little bit more expensive, but there's nothing better for you to spend your money on than a health-promoting diet. And it tastes so good, you'll only need to use a small amount. Avocado oil is another monounsaturated fat that's rich in healthy EFAs.

Canola oil is also monounsaturated, but it's highly processed. It's best to use canola oil only very occasionally. If you love chips and have to have them, buy chips fried in canola oil rather than in unsaturated oils (vegetable or nut oils) or hydrogenated oils that show up on labels as a "partially hydrogenated" oil. (Better yet, bake your own.) Unsaturated oils, also called polyunsaturated, are most likely rancid by the time you open the bottle to use them, so you can imagine how far gone they are when they've been sitting on the kitchen shelf for a while or when they're exposed to high temperatures during cooking.

In general, refined oils such as canola oil are put through intensive processing. Toxic chemicals that leave behind toxic residues are used to extract these oils from their vegetable, nut, or seed of origin. Sometimes synthetic preservatives are added back in to replace the natural antioxidants destroyed in processing.

❧ ORGANIC FOODS ARE A KEY TO HORMONE BALANCE

Organic foods are grown in uncontaminated soil without pesticides of any kind (including herbicides, fungicides, and insecticides), without chemical fertilizers and additives, and without sewage sludge. Also, they are not genetically engineered. Organic farmers have found over the years that healthy soil produces healthy plants, which contain an abundance of natural substances that allow them to better resist diseases and pests.

Fruits and vegetables that are conventionally grown are low in nutrients, hybridized, sprayed, and fertilized with all manner of xenohormonic pesticides and other poisonous compounds. Nonorganic farming leaves soil depleted of the minerals it needs to produce healthy, pest-resistant crops. Those hardy plants that can be eked out of this used-up soil need plenty of xenoestrogenic fertilizers and pesticides. The hybridization of crops— which is what makes those uniformly large, flawless-looking veggies you see in the supermarket produce section—means further exhaustion of nutrient content.

Our food crops today have half the nutrients of crops grown a century ago, and we consume less food than our ancestors (who spent much of the day at hard physical labor). Factor in generally poor digestion and the fact that we tend to cook the nutrients out of our vegetables, and add in the large amounts of processed food that have replaced whole foods, and you have a setup for poor health: the low nutritional intake of the average person in an industrialized culture.

Meats and dairy products are even more tainted by conventional farming methods. Enormous factory farms raise cattle and pigs jammed into pens that deny them exercise and sunlight. Their feed falls far short of being anything you'd want to put in your own belly. If you are what you eat, you're also what whatever you eat eats. In some instances cattle are fed old newspapers that other cattle have urinated on, or a mishmash of oils, waste from crops, and unsalable parts of their slaughtered brethren. On such a dietary regimen, livestock are generally unable to fight off infections and are maintained on a steady diet of antibiotics to keep them alive. Then they are given hormones to artificially fatten them up. Range-raised cattle, on the other hand, are naturally lean. The fats found in the meat of a cow that has been grazed in open pasture are stable and saturated, whereas the meat of cattle raised in factory farms contains a bizarre not-found-in-nature conglomeration of polyunsaturated and saturated fats, chemicals, and hormones. Conventional chickens and dairy cattle are raised under similar conditions, and their eggs and milk contain the poisonous stuff they are fed.

Xenohormones (e.g., pesticides) contained in the foods (such as grains) fed to livestock are concentrated in the fat, which means you're getting a relatively potent dose when you eat fatty meat. The bottom line here is that whenever possible, use only organic meats, eggs, and dairy products. If you're on a tight budget and can only afford to buy some of your foods as organics, these are the ones you should choose. Look for free-range, hormone-free and drug-free eggs, dairy, meats, and chicken.

If you do drink milk, be sure to get it from cows that are not given bovine growth hormone, known as rBGH, which is used to force the cows' bodies into producing higher quantities of milk. Milk from cows given rBGH has higher levels of pus (an indication of infection) in their milk, and we really have no idea of what long-term consequences of its use may be. Milk that is free of rBGH should state that on the container, or there may be a notice posted in the dairy section giving you the information.

❖ LET VEGETABLES BE YOUR DRUGSTORE

Phytochemicals are plant compounds, and many of them have health-supporting effects on the body. It's estimated that there are more than ten thousand of these compounds in the plants we eat. Phytoestrogens are one type of phytochemical that has a variety of weak estrogen-like activities. They compete for estrogen receptors throughout the body, helping to block the effects of excess estrogen. Soybeans are the most celebrated source of phytoestrogens these days, and they also contain compounds that are beneficial in fighting cancer. If you eat a variety of fresh vegetables and have soy products a few times a week, you'll reap the benefits of these natural estrogens. There are many herbs, including black cohosh, licorice root, anise, and fennel that contain phytoestrogens.

Please be wary of all the hype around soy. Although it does contain compounds that can help balance your hormones, it is far from a magic hormone balance solution. Soy contains compounds that block the absorption of needed nutrients like zinc and will disable enzymes your body needs to access other nutrients. It directly blocks thyroid function and protein absorption. Many people are allergic to soy products, and women who are extremely sensitive to estrogens of any kind may react negatively to them.

The traditional Asian processing methods used to make fermented soy products—tofu, tempeh, and miso—get rid of most of the toxins and make the beneficial phytochemicals more available to the body. Tofu and tempeh are a nearly complete protein and as such are an excellent alternative to meat in a balanced meal. Miso stirred into hot water with a strip of kombu or nori (seaweeds) makes a satisfying soup base or beverage. To offset the negative side of soy, Dr. David Zava recommends eating fermented soy products and tofu as the Asians do, with a protein such as fish and a rich mineral source such as the seaweeds.

Soy milks and soy protein powders aren't in the same league as the fermented soy products, so use them sparingly. There's a good chance that the soybean toxins are more concentrated in these products, and they may do you more harm than good over the long haul.

Please don't eat soy three times a day or even every day. That undermines your goal of balance. Aim for two or three times a week and get the rest of your phytochemicals from a wide variety of fresh fruits and vegetables.

Some phytochemicals are also potent cancer fighters, and this is why people who eat lots of vegetables have much lower rates of all types of cancer. The box on page 308 gives you a detailed look at some known anticancer vegetables and how they protect you.

❧ SOME PHYTOCHEMICALS FOUND IN ❧ FOODS AND THEIR ANTICANCER ACTIONS

Plant	Chemical	Action in body
Broccoli	Sulforaphane	Removes carcinogens from cells by boosting enzyme activity
	Phenethyl isothiocyanate	Binds to enzymes which otherwise would bind carcinogens to DNA
Broccoli, cauliflower, cabbage	Indole-3 carbinol	Helps a precursor to estrogen break up into a benign rather than a cancer-causing form
Citrus fruits	Flavonoids	Prevents cancer-causing hormones from latching onto a cell
Onions and garlic	Allylic sulfide	Detoxifies carcinogens
Hot peppers	Capsaicin	Keeps toxic molecules from attaching to DNA
Soybeans	Genistein	Prevents growth of new blood vessels to cancer cells, which are needed for tumor growth
Tomatoes	p-coumaric acid chlorogenic acid	Both disrupt the chemical wedding between two common chemicals in cells—a union that can produce carcinogens, e.g., nitrosamine

❧ FIBER IS THE GREAT EQUALIZER AND DETOXIFIER

Plant cell walls are our food sources of fiber. Fiber is not just a rough broom that makes bowel movements easier; it also serves as a source of important nutrients for the friendly bacteria that live in our digestive tracts.

Cellulose, found in most plant foods, binds water in the digestive tract, which makes for easier and more frequent elimination. Other varieties of fiber form gels within which excess dietary cholesterol is trapped (and so not absorbed by the body). The types of fiber found in beans and around the moist inner layer of seeds have potent cholesterol-lowering effects. Fiber known as lignin is broken down into compounds that are protective against cancer.

A whole panoply of diseases has been connected to low-fiber diets. High blood pressure, heart disease, varicose veins, diverticulitis (painful pouchings along the large intestine), colon cancer, irritable bowel syndrome, constipation, Crohn's disease (severe chronic inflammation of the colon), and hemorrhoids (varicose veins in the rectum) are a few of the conditions that can be prevented with a diet rich in fiber.

Constipation means that wastes sit longer in your colon, and that means greater reabsorption of xenoestrogens from waste and a greater toxic estrogen load. If you have a bowel movement at least once a day, you are eliminating toxins from your system rather than reabsorbing them.

A high-fiber diet is also important for the maintenance of "friendly" colon bacteria like *Lactobacillus*. Friendly bacteria counter the overgrowth of toxin-producing bacteria and yeasts. (We'll talk more about yeast overgrowth a little later in this chapter.)

A plant-eating animal our size living in the wild would take in 30 to 90 g of fiber a day. The average human gets only about 10 g a day. Most humans maintain their best health on at least 30 g of fiber a day. If you eat whole foods, that will be easy. And here's an added bonus: On a high-fiber diet you'll feel more satiated with less food. You'll eat less and probably lose a few pounds.

If you change your diet to focus more on whole foods and still are not having a bowel movement daily, you may want to add supplemental psyllium. You can try Metamucil or other store brands, but avoid those containing sweeteners and food coloring. You can also buy psyllium in bulk at your health food store. Stir one to three teaspoons into a large glass of water and drink it immediately, or stir it into a medium-size glass of water and follow it with another glass of water. You can also use rice bran and mix it into your food.

❖ IDENTIFY AND ELIMINATE PROBLEM FOODS

When Jennifer first went to see Dr. Hanley, she was a successful personal trainer who exercised daily, used supplements, and followed a strict vegetarian diet. Upon closer examination Dr. Hanley saw that inside the well-muscled, energetic body that sat on her examining table, there was a lot going wrong. Her skin was pale and blotchy, and she seemed exhausted and terribly short of breath, with an awful rattling cough.

"I don't know what to do anymore," she told Dr. Hanley at their first appointment. "I've had asthma since I finished school five years ago. I never had it before that. It was right about the time I got married and became a vegan that I started wheezing a little bit during my morning runs. Since then it's gotten worse and worse. Now it flares up from just walking down the street. I've grown so dependent on my inhalers, and they're not even working that well anymore—I have to take twice as much to breathe easier."

Twice a year like clockwork Jennifer would come down with bronchitis, and during her most recent bout, she had had to make a middle-of-the-night trip to the emergency room because of a severe asthma attack. She had been through an expensive series of tests to discover that she was allergic to most pollens, dog and cat dander, and dust mites. Eczema, depression, bloating, constipation, and hemorrhoids plagued her as well. It was getting harder and harder for her to get out of bed in the morning, and she couldn't seem to get going without two cups of strong coffee and another in the afternoon. Her conventional doctor wanted to put her on powerful steroid drugs and Prozac, but Jennifer was determined to find another way.

When Dr. Hanley asked her about her diet, she discovered that Jennifer had been eating some vegetables, legumes, and fruit, but her main food was wheat. With every meal she would eat bread or bagels. Sometimes all she would eat until dinnertime was wheat. Dr. Hanley then asked about her lifestyle in general, and gathered that Jennifer was very stressed, never allowing herself a rest from her responsibilities in her work and in her marriage. She was the breadwinner in the family, putting her husband through graduate school. Even when her asthma was acting up she taught exercise classes and did her own workouts. She tried to keep up with coffee and inhalers, both of which made her jittery.

When Dr. Hanley recommended that she start adding some animal protein back into her diet, Jennifer chuckled. "My husband would never allow that. He won't allow any eggs, dairy, or meat in the house. I'd have to sneak out and have it somewhere else." She was desperate to feel better, though, and Dr. Hanley convinced her to try cutting out wheat for several weeks, focusing instead on whole foods, and Jennifer agreed to go out for fish two to three times a week at lunchtime. She also agreed to cut out caffeine, and she went home with digestive enzymes, betaine hydrochloride (HCl), quercetin, a B vitamin complex, and natural hydrocortisone to take daily with meals along with her other supplements. (You'll learn more about all of these supplements later in this chapter and about hydrocortisone in chapter 17.)

Six weeks later Jennifer returned, looking like a different person. The knitted brow, the patchy dry skin and shortness of breath were gone. Her energy seemed entirely different—more even and sustained. Her nasal allergies and itchy eyes were all but gone, and she could breathe much more freely. Her face had lost its swollen look. "Even the cats that live in my house don't bother me anymore," she told Dr. Hanley. "I can let them sleep on my face if I want. I've started doing yoga and meditating more. I feel as if you've given me a second chance at life."

Jennifer's wheat-based diet had caused a general state of inflammation throughout her body, and she had developed multiple allergies as her immune system lost track of which substances, from pollens and dust to foods and pollution, were harmless to her body and which needed to be attacked. The added effects of undue stress had made her airways hyperreactive to any stimulus. Several years of this had exhausted her energy reserves and she had made the problem worse by using caffeine and stimulant inhalers to muscle through the day.

When she fell off the wagon on a vacation and started eating wheat several times a day again, all of her symptoms returned with a vengeance. She kicked it by abstaining completely from wheat for six months, and now she can eat wheat once or twice a week without problems.

Food allergy is not something the average physician knows anything about. In fact most consider it hocus-pocus in spite of the fact that they are unable to cure the many illnesses caused by food allergies, such as irritable bowel syndrome, Crohn's disease, colitis, eczema, acne, fibromyalgia, arthritis, and depression. This attitude comes as no surprise, because most are taught virtually nothing about nutrition in medical school. Food allergies generally aren't the kind that quickly make your nose run or your eyes itch the way pollens do, or the kind where you break out in hives and swell up and have to be rushed to the emergency room. These *immediate* or acute allergic reactions are easy to spot and to connect to specific allergens, like pollens or dust mites or bee stings. Common foods that cause immediate allergic reactions are strawberries, seafood, peanuts, and dairy products. It's not uncommon for children to have immediate allergies to foods, but they usually outgrow them.

The food allergies that Jennifer suffered from are of the *delayed* variety. The response is slow and sustained and difficult to pinpoint without eliminating potentially problematic foods to see if symptoms improve. Symptoms tend to be diffuse and come on slowly, after many years of daily intake of the foods you're sensitive to. Food allergy can affect digestion, muscles, joints, emotional well-being, energy levels, skin, lungs, and water balance, causing headache, rashes, muscle and joint aches, fatigue, hay fever, asthma, malabsorption of nutrients, and indigestion. It's amazing how many people struggle through every day feeling generally ill and tired, thinking that that's just the way life is and that they have to get used to it.

❧ THE ELIMINATION DIET

If you want to feel your absolute best, you need to identify and eliminate foods you're sensitive to. Doing so changes your body chemistry dramatically in ways you have to experience to believe. You can begin by keeping a detailed diet journal for two weeks, then make a list of all of the foods you eat every day or more than five times a week. These are probably foods you cannot imagine going a single day without, the foods that satisfy your most urgent cravings. A typical list of these foods might include wheat products, corn, citrus fruits, milk products, nightshade vegetables (tomatoes, potatoes, red and green peppers, cayenne pepper, or eggplant), peanuts, coffee, eggs, or beef—the most commonly allergenic foods. If your most commonly eaten foods are processed, like cookies or candy, figure out the main ingredients. (Most contain wheat and dairy.) If you've had irritable bowel syndrome—alternating constipation and diarrhea with painful gas and bloating—you're probably allergic to dairy products.

Celiac disease, often mistaken for Crohn's disease, is an allergic reaction to gluten-containing grains. Gluten is a component of many grains including wheat, oats, rye, barley, quinoa, spelt, and amaranth. If you're allergic to wheat there's a good chance you're also allergic to the other gluten-containing grains. You can replace them with rice, corn (some people may be allergic to this as well), buckwheat, millet, soy, potato flour, tapioca, or arrowroot products. You should find many alternatives at your health food store.

Preservatives and additives are very irritating to some people; look out for nitrates, sulfites, benzoates, red and yellow food dyes, MSG (monosodium glutamate), BHT (butylated hydroxytoluene), and BHA (butylated hydroxyanisole), or anything else that sounds like something made in a chemical laboratory rather than by Mother Nature.

Be very careful to eliminate all potential sources of allergenic foods, which may be hidden in vitamins and processed foods. In fact, it's best if you eliminate processed foods entirely during your elimination diet.

Once you've made your list of likely suspects, it's time to eliminate these foods completely from your diet for at least two weeks. Of the foods you are eating, avoid eating any one food every day during the two weeks, or you may create a new sensitivity to that food. Continue to record *everything* you eat and how you are feeling.

Keep careful track of your responses as you go. During the first three days of an elimination diet, you may feel terrible. Don't be surprised if you have powerful withdrawal symptoms. When we have an allergic response to food the body releases mood- and energy-enhancing chemicals such as adrenaline to fight back, so we tend to become hooked on the foods we are most sensitive to. Also, as you eliminate allergenic foods your body will quickly seize the opportunity to detoxify itself, causing symptoms such as headaches and even skin rashes. If you are allergic to the foods you have eliminated, you'll start to feel very good after a few days.

At the end of the two weeks, reintroduce the suspected foods one at a time. No more than one food should be reintroduced every 24 hours, and if you get a reaction, wait another 24 hours before reintroducing another new food. Continue to record all symptoms you experience. Troublesome foods may cause symptoms such as rapid or uneven heart rhythms, sleepiness or fatigue, mental lethargy, stomach cramps, bloating, gas, diarrhea, constipation, headache, chills, sweats, flushing, and achiness.

When you have reintroduced all of your suspect foods and identified those that caused a reaction, eliminate them from your diet for at least two months. If your symptoms were severe, eliminate them for six months. Reintroduce them by eating them first thing in the morning and waiting at least an hour before eating anything else. If you still have a reaction, wait six months and try again. Eventually you will be able to eat the offending foods occasionally, but if you start eating them every day again you'll probably become sensitive to them again. For people who tend to be sensitive to foods, it's always a good idea to rotate the foods you eat and avoid eating any one food every day.

✤ GOOD HORMONE BALANCE BEGINS IN THE DIGESTIVE TRACT

If you suffer from indigestion, heartburn, gas, bloating, or constipation, it's a good bet that your digestive tract needs a little help. And that does *not* mean taking Tums or Tagamet. In some cases, all it takes is eating whole foods and avoiding food allergens. Others need extra support.

Heartburn isn't caused by excess stomach acid—it is

caused when food is too slowly digested and escapes back into the esophagus. Because it's now mixed with acid, it burns uncomfortably. A meal very high in fat will slow digestion way down. That's why fried foods cause heartburn. In a large percentage of those who are popping Pepto-Bismol tablets and Zantac to relieve their symptoms, the problem is actually too *little* stomach acid. If the acid-secreting cells in your stomach aren't doing the job right, food sits around in your stomach too long. The acidity of the mass of digested food in your stomach eventually gives the signal for it to pass into the small intestine. If there isn't enough acid, it takes much longer to move food out of the stomach.

If you have chronic digestive problems that include belching, bloating, a heavy feeling in the gut, or heartburn, you probably aren't making enough stomach acid. For some, simply stimulating acid secretion by drinking a glass of water a half hour before eating helps. A tablespoon of apple cider vinegar in one-third of a cup of water, or 500 mg vitamin C powder in water just before a meal acidifies the stomach as well. You may want to try a supplement called betaine hydrochloride (HCl). It's made of the same acids your stomach makes. Take 2 to 20 grains (or follow directions on the bottle), building up the dose slowly. If you feel a burning in your stomach after using them, you've taken too much. Don't use betaine HCl during attacks of heartburn or if you have an ulcer.

Your pancreas secretes enzymes into the small intestine as food passes through it. These enzymes work along with enzymes naturally present in raw foods to break down proteins, fats, and carbohydrates into their most basic components (amino acids, free fatty acids, and glucose). Vitamins and minerals are also freed for absorption during this process. If the pancreas isn't making enough enzymes, that means that food isn't completely broken down or efficiently absorbed. You may notice a lot of undigested food in your stools if this is the case.

Some digestive problems are caused by lactose intolerance. Lactose, a protein found in milk, can't be broken down in those with lactose intolerance because their bodies don't make the enzyme lactase. Lactose molecules pass through the system undigested and are fermented by bacteria in the large intestine. This causes gas, bloating, and diarrhea. If you're not making the enzymes you need, this is what happens as undigested bits of food reach your large intestine.

You can try a digestive enzyme supplement that contains protease, amylase, lipase, cellulose, and lactase (if you eat dairy products). Some enzyme supplements also contain papaya and pineapple enzymes (papain and bromelain). Take them after meals according to the directions on the container.

❖ CANDIDIASIS IS FOR REAL

We spoke briefly about "friendly" bacteria on page 310. These bacteria, also called probiotics, manufacture some of the B vitamins and fatty acids, and they are your defense against yeast (*Candida albicans*) overgrowth and an almost infinite variety of other hostile bacterial and viral invaders. Candida grows naturally in our small and large intestines, and is harmless as long as balance is maintained. On a steady diet of processed sugars and flours—the preferred foods of yeast—it can grow out of control, resulting in vaginal and gastrointestinal yeast overgrowth (candidiasis). If you've had to take a lot of antibiotics in your lifetime, your risk of having this problem is much greater. Antibiotics kill all bacteria, good and bad, allowing yeast to grow unfettered. Anytime you have to use antibiotics, follow them with a two-week course of probiotic supplements, which contain friendly bacteria that help keep candida in check. You can find probiotic supplements at your health food store in the refrigerated section.

Most women know that vaginal yeast infections are very unpleasant, but yeast overgrowth in the digestive system is equally problematic. It creates inflammation and releases toxins into the bloodstream that can cause myriad symptoms. Much like those caused by food allergy, the symptoms of candidiasis tend to be generalized and not severe enough to stop you in your tracks. Fatigue, rashes, irritable bowel, aches and pains, and allergies can be related to yeast overgrowth. Candidiasis predisposes us to food allergy. Severe PMS with depression, mood swings, and fluid retention, irregular periods, infertility, and endometriosis have been linked to this state of imbalance as well.

Conventional medical doctors often pooh-pooh candidiasis, but they are likely to resort to antidepressant or antianxiety drugs combined with potent stomach acid-blocking drugs when faced with the spectrum of problems presented by this illness, because they don't know how else to treat it. Those drugs only make the problem worse, and over time severe illness and debilitation can result.

Some health care professionals will prescribe powerful antifungal drugs to treat candidiasis, but it makes sense to first try a more low-key approach such as boosting your immune system and supporting your digestive system. The pharmaceutical antifungals have many potential side effects and can be hard on the liver and kidneys.

Another common strategy for treating candida overgrowth is a very strict diet that eliminates every type of food and drink that candida loves to feed on (sugars) as well as foods that aggravate your immune system's overreaction to the overgrowth. These foods include anything made with yeasts such as bread and beer, and pickled foods such as wine and cheese.

If you are diagnosed with candidiasis, or even suspect that you have it, the best cure is a good defense. That means supporting your digestive system by taking probiotics, eating whole foods high in fiber, and cutting way back on refined carbohydrates and sugar. Live-culture yogurt and kefir are good sources of friendly bacteria. Check the labels to be sure they contain live cultures. Buy the plain unsweetened yogurt and add your own fruit to avoid the large amount of sugar hiding in the presweetened types. If you buy probiotic supplements, look for them in the refrigerated case of your health food store and keep them refrigerated when you get home. Take them as directed on the container, on an empty stomach.

A lifetime of nutritional deficiencies, overeating, toxic foods, and frequent antibiotic use is at the root of the majority of food allergy and digestive problems. The cells that make digestive acids and enzymes have hard work to do, and when they don't get the nutrients they need to handle the large amounts of food in the typical American diet, they can only hold up for so long without getting exhausted or damaged.

The same goes for the delicate lining of the small intestines. In the twists and turns of this long tube, nutrients are absorbed through millions of tiny finger-like strands called villi. Poor nutrition, overuse of non-steroidal anti-inflammatory drugs (NSAIDs) such as aspirin and ibuprofen, antibiotics, and infection all contribute to a condition called leaky gut, which Dr. Hanley and many other alternative health care professionals believe is epidemic in the United States. Microscopic holes are eroded in the intestinal lining, allowing toxins to escape into the blood and blocking the ability of the villi to send nutrients in. When undigested food particles and toxins enter the bloodstream, the immune system attacks.

Leaky gut is probably the most common cause of food allergy and arthritis. Healing a leaky gut involves all the steps we've described: whole foods diet, elimination of problem foods, and drinking plenty of water. You can also take 500 mg up to four times a day of glutamine, an amino acid that is the preferred fuel of the intestinal lining. Eat plenty of deep water fish and fresh vegetables for their anti-inflammatory oils.

✤ THE PREMENOPAUSE SUPPLEMENT PROGRAM

Almost everyone can benefit from a good multivitamin. Even if your diet is generally healthy, think of it as insurance against nutritional deficiencies, environmental toxins, and daily stress.

If you can't tolerate multivitamins, don't feel pressured into forcing yourself to take them. Your body has its own profound wisdom, and it is more important to trust that than any generic nutrition advice. Many multivitamins are quite contaminated with manufacturing by-products, binders, and fillers, and you may be reacting to them. Often it is the odor of the B vitamins that are the culprit. You can test that by smelling a B-complex supplement. If the smell makes you recoil, try taking your vitamins separately or find a brand that doesn't contain yeast, which often has an objectionable odor. For example, you can take a good antioxidant and a good multimineral supplement. Have a B-complex handy and give it a "sniff test" occasionally. If the odor isn't repulsive to you, take some; you probably need it. Some people can't tolerate vitamin C. If that's you, find an antioxidant without vitamin C.

Vitamins and minerals come in just about every form imaginable. If you don't like swallowing tablets or capsules you can also get vitamins in liquid and powder form. You can also inhale them, put them under your tongue, and rub them on your skin. Experiment and find what works best for you.

Choosing a multivitamin can be difficult because there are so many out there, but you can refer to the section that follows as a general guideline. In general it's best to avoid the supermarket and drugstore vitamins because they tend to have low dosages—check the label. Make sure that if you're taking a tablet it dissolves. One way to test that is to drop it into a glass of water. If it takes more than fifteen minutes to dissolve, find another brand.

❖ VITAMINS

When it comes to vitamin dosages, you may need to experiment to find what works best for you personally. You should be able to find a good multivitamin that contains all of these nutrients in the recommended ranges.

Beta-carotene/Carotenoids

Take 10,000 to 15,000 IU daily. Carotenoids are powerful antioxidants found in colorful fruits and vegetables, especially the yellow, orange, and red ones. Beta-carotene is an important carotenoid. Some beta-carotene is converted to vitamin A in the body. Unlike vitamin A, beta-carotene is water-soluble, which means that any that isn't needed is flushed out in the urine. Always take beta-carotene in mixed carotenoids and with a mix of other antioxidants that includes vitamin E, because there is some evidence that taken alone it can be harmful. Remember, in nature, beta-carotene is always found packaged with hundreds of other ingredients. Beta-carotene is found in higher concentrations in the ovaries than anywhere else in a woman's body. This may be an indication that it's protective. Eat your carrots! Your best bet is to find a multivitamin that contains a mix of carotenoids.

Vitamin A

Take 5,000 to 10,000 IU daily (in addition to the carotenoids). This antioxidant is fat-soluble, and reserves can be stored in the liver for long periods. This also means that it can build up to toxic levels if more than 10,000 IU is taken daily for a long period of time. Vitamin A helps your body fight infections and speed wound healing. If you're not pregnant, you can take up to 50,000 IU for up to a week if you're fighting an infection. Please don't be scared away from vitamin A if you're pregnant. Adequate amounts are essential for a healthy baby. Just don't overdo it. The generally accepted maximum for a pregnant woman is 10,000 IU daily. Fish, meat, and poultry are naturally rich in vitamin A.

B Vitamins

The following B vitamins should be taken daily.

Biotin: 100 to 300 mcg (micrograms)
Choline: 50 to 100 mg

Folic acid/folate/folacin: 400 to 800 mcg
Inositol: 150 to 300 mg
Niacin (B3): 20 to 25 mg
Pantothenic acid (B5): 50 to 100 mg
Pyridoxine (B6): 25 to 50 mg
Riboflavin (B2): 25 to 50 mg
Thiamine (B1): 25 to 50 mg
Vitamin B12: 1,000 to 2,000 mcg

Stress levels tend to be high for the average premenopausal woman. Whether you are working, raising children or both, your reserves can get drained quickly. B vitamins are an important part of your stress-buffering system. If you're under more stress than usual, you may want to add an extra B complex to your multivitamin for a little insurance.

The B vitamins play multiple roles in brain function, mood regulation, the transformation of food into energy within the cells, and neutralizing of a toxic by-product of protein metabolism called homocysteine. High levels of homocysteine are a newly emerging and very substantial risk factor for heart disease—it directly damages the walls of blood vessels.

The B vitamins, especially vitamin B6, play an important role as enzyme cofactors that transform one hormone to another. A deficiency of vitamin B6 and folic acid can contribute to cervical hyperplasia, and folic acid deficiency is also strongly implicated in colon cancer. Folic acid deficiency during pregnancy, even very early on, can cause neural tube defects, so this is a "must" vitamin for any woman who even has the possibility of becoming pregnant.

Pantothenic acid and inositol play pivotal roles in blood sugar regulation and balance, allergy control, arthritis, and energy production in the cells.

Unless you're treating a specific health problem, the B vitamins should always be taken together (called a B complex) as just taking one can cause imbalances of the others. The misguided practice of stripping the B vitamins out of wheat flour in the refining practice and then adding back a few of them undoubtedly contributes to a variety of health problems—yet another reason to be sure you're eating whole grains.

Whole grains, meat, and liver in particular are rich sources of B vitamins, but they are also found in most other foods in smaller amounts. (Since the liver concentrates toxins, please only eat liver from organic livestock.) It is difficult to get adequate amounts of vitamin B12 when you are a vegetarian, so be sure to supplement it if you don't eat meat or dairy products. Sometimes just taking a supplement of betaine HCl increases stomach acid enough so that the conversion of B12 in the stomach can be made. Since the symptoms of B12 deficiency can take a long time to appear, it's best to be on the safe side. If you suspect you have low stomach acid, try a betaine HCl supplement. (See page 317 for a discussion on digestion.)

Vitamin C

Take 500 to 1,000 mg daily. This superantioxidant nutrient has been making news for decades, since Linus Pauling began researching its amazing immunity-boosting effects. Vitamin C is also an important component of collagen, the basic building block of connective tissue. It's water-soluble, so you eliminate what you don't need. When you're sick or stressed, you go through vitamin C at a much faster rate. It's a good idea to keep a bottle of buffered vitamin C (either esterified or as calcium or magnesium ascorbate) around so that you can take more when you're coming down with something or are under the proverbial gun. You can take up to 10,000 mg per day when you're under a lot of stress or getting sick. If it gives you diarrhea, take a lower dose. Good food sources include citrus fruits, tomatoes, potatoes, mangoes, kiwis, and red peppers. Vitamin C is destroyed by time and heat, another good reason to eat plenty of fresh, raw foods.

Vitamin D

Take 100 to 400 IU daily. Vitamin D is really more like a hormone than a vitamin, and it has multiple roles in the body. We make some vitamin D when we go out into the sunshine, but a little extra is a good idea, especially for women and especially in the winter. If you live in a rainy northern climate or are a vegetarian take the higher doses. If you can, spend at least 15 minutes a day outside, without sunblock or sunglasses. There's a lot we don't understand about vitamin D, but we do know that it interacts with calcium and phosphorus to build strong, healthy bones.

Vitamin D is fat-soluble and can build up to toxic levels if high doses are taken for long. Fish is the best source of vitamin D, and cow's milk (though generally not recommended unless you're a baby cow) is fortified with it.

Vitamin E

Take 200 to 400 IU daily. The many roles of this fat-soluble antioxidant are the subject of a great deal of research these days. It stops free radicals from damaging cells and repairs other "spent" antioxidants and B vitamins. It's a natural blood thinner, relieves fibrocystic breasts and edema (accumulation of excess fluid), and strengthens blood vessel walls. There is an abundance of research showing that vitamin E is powerfully protective against heart attacks and strokes. It is an important part of a PMS supplement regimen. Vitamin E is found in whole grains, vegetables, and nuts. Our diets of vitamin E-deficient, refined carbohydrates have created a virtual epidemic of vitamin E deficiency. Vitamin E is destroyed by food processing and light. This is a vitamin that almost everyone can benefit from in supplement form.

❖ MINERALS

The passage of minerals in and out of cells is a delicately balanced operation, dependent on the health of the membrane around each cell. Levels of estrogen that are too high coupled with synthetic progestins actually impair the action of cell membranes, while natural progesterone heals cell membranes and allows normal mineral balance to be restored. A daily combination supplement should include boron, calcium, chromium, copper, magnesium, manganese, selenium, vanadyl sulfate, and zinc.

Boron

Take 1 to 5 mg daily. Although we don't know the exact mechanisms, we know that this mineral plays a role in the maintenance of healthy bones.

Calcium

Take 300 mg daily with magnesium.

Calcium is well known for its role as a bone and tooth builder, and that's the role of 99 percent of the calcium in the body. Calcium can't get into bone without the help of many other substances, most notable magnesium and vitamin D. The 1 percent left over is an indispensable player in nerve conduction, muscle contraction, heartbeat and blood pressure regulation, clotting of blood, and functioning of the thyroid gland. Contrary to what dairy industry ads would have you believe, milk is a poor source of calcium because it lacks the magnesium necessary to get it into the bone. Milk also promotes heart disease. Both Dr. Lee and Dr. Hanley strongly recommend avoiding milk. Tofu (soybean curd), black-eyed peas, leafy green vegetables, and broccoli are good sources of calcium in the diet.

Chromium

Take 200 to 400 mcg daily. This trace mineral keeps blood sugars steady so that you can fight off cravings for sugar and refined flour. It also helps manufacture needed nutrients like cholesterol and fatty acids. It's found naturally in mushrooms, beef, beets, liver, and whole grains. Low-fat, processed food diets often result in chromium deficiency.

Copper

Take 1 to 5 mg daily. Copper has many roles in the body, including wound healing; transport of oxygen through the blood (it's a component of the body's oxygen-carrying molecule hemoglobin); and maintaining the integrity of nerves, skin, and bones. Seafood, beans, almonds, whole grains, and green leafy vegetables are good sources of this mineral.

Estrogen-dominant women should be aware that long-term treatment with synthetic drug contraceptives (pills, shots), estrogen, and progestins has the side effect of causing loss of zinc and retention of copper. Both act as coenzymes involved with manufacturing neurotransmitters in the brain. An imbalance of these two minerals can lead to mood swings and make handling stress difficult. Chronic copper excess can cause psychotic episodes. Dr. Lee believes that this imbalance, first noted by hormone researcher Dr. Ellen Grant, is what can tip the scale and turn mild PMS irritation into rage.

Magnesium

Take 400 to 600 mg (chelated) at bedtime daily. This mineral is involved in just about every aspect of our physiology. It makes up .05 percent of our body weight and is incorporated into bones as well as being distributed throughout our other tissues. Calcium and magnesium need each other to fulfill their roles. Intravenous magnesium has been used to treat heart arrhythmias, high blood pressure, heart failure, asthma, fibromyalgia, and chronic fatigue syndrome with great success. It's also an effective laxative taken orally in higher doses. Most Americans are sorely deficient in magnesium, which is found in nuts, seeds, figs, corn, apples, soybeans, milk, and wheat germ.

Magnesium plays a role in most hormone actions. Many migraine sufferers find relief simply by taking 400 to 800 mg magnesium daily.

If you have asthma, chronic muscle cramps, or high blood pressure, or are at high risk of osteoporosis or heart disease, take 400 mg in the morning and evening for a total of 800 mg. Don't take enough to cause diarrhea. This is a supplement that can help almost everyone.

Manganese

Take 5 to 20 mg daily. The B vitamins and vitamin C need manganese to do their jobs. This mineral also helps the thyroid gland and ovaries make their hormones and participates in the synthesis of carbohydrates, fatty acids, cholesterol, bone, and protein. It's an important mineral for hormone balance as well as for prevention of heart disease and diabetes. Egg yolks, green vegetables, seeds, whole grains, and nuts contain generous amounts of manganese.

Selenium

Take 100 to 200 mcg daily. This mineral behaves like an antioxidant in the body and has a long list of other important jobs. Selenium and vitamin E work together to prevent the oxidation of unsaturated fats in the bloodstream. Prostaglandins can't be produced without selenium. It also plays a role in cellular energy production and is a powerful anticancer substance. Selenium is also a powerful antiviral substance and can be used in higher doses to ward off colds and flu and to prevent herpes outbreaks. You can take 200 mcg (*micrograms*) two or three times daily for up to a week as a preventive. High levels of selenium over time (more than 1 mg daily for more than two weeks) can be toxic, so don't overdo it.

Vanadyl sulfate

Take 5 to 10 mg daily. Vanadium, taken in the form of vanadyl sulfate, is another blood sugar balancing mineral that works cooperatively with chromium and enhances the process of shuttling glucose (sugar) from the blood into the cells.

Zinc

Take 15 to 30 mg daily. As noted above, a deficiency of zinc combined with an excess of copper can lead to severe mood disturbances and imbalance. Soy products directly block the absorption of zinc, which is one reason we don't recommend eating them every day.

Zinc is also an important cofactor in hormonal metabolism and has jobs to do in almost every tissue in the body. Although zinc is present in trace amounts in most foods, it is most abundant in meat, poultry, fish, and dairy products. Vegetarians take note: You'll definitely need to supplement this mineral if you are strictly vegan.

Note that iron is not included among the recommended minerals. Unless you have documented iron deficiency or anemia, there's no reason for you to take extra iron. An excess of iron can be very harmful, sparking the formation of free radicals. However, if you have heavy bleeding during your menstrual period for more than two months, it's a good idea to get a blood test to check your iron levels.

❖ OTHER SUPPLEMENTS FOR HORMONE BALANCE

Apart from vitamins and minerals, there are other supplements you can take to help you balance your hormones. Borage oil and evening primrose oil contain essential fatty acids that work as natural anti-inflammatories. Used before and during the onset of PMS, these oils can help ease symptoms. Take according to the instructions on the bottle. Get a brand that supplies the equivalent of 300 mg GLA oils daily.

Quercetin is a bioflavonoid that has potent antioxidant and antiallergy effects. Found in nutritious foods like green apples and onions, it's being intently studied for its potential as a heart disease and cancer preventive. Use 250 to 500 mg three times a day, between meals.

Selenium, elderberry, echinacea, and antioxidants are used to prevent colds and flu from getting the best of you every winter—or to fight off any infection. Take extra selenium (200 mcg more than recommended in your daily vitamins, two or three times daily with meals); elderberry (which contains powerful antioxidants; follow directions on the container); vitamin C (up to 10,000 mg in divided doses in a buffered form); vitamin E (800 IU) and beta-carotene (25,000 IU). This combination of nutrients supports your immune system so that it can more quickly conquer whatever bug has taken hold of you. You can take these supplements when you know your immune system is compromised, such as when you are traveling, when you feel a cold or flu coming on, or when you have a cold or flu. Don't take them for more than two weeks at a time.

Echinacea is an immune-stimulating herb that can be useful when taken at the first signs of a cold or flu (follow instructions on the container). It doesn't seem to help much once a cold or flu has taken hold.

❧ IT'S UP TO YOU

We are all at this very moment being bombarded by toxins and stresses. Even under the best of circumstances, our foods are not as nutritious as they need to be to support us. We have to recognize the weaknesses of our modern lifestyle and do what we can to fill the gaps. This doesn't mean becoming obsessed with our food and our supplements or abandoning our exciting but stressful lives. What it does mean is that we should do the best we can to adequately nourish ourselves and protect ourselves from things that make us sick.

Our bodies need real food, real exercise, and respect. Young women can temporarily get away with treating their bodies with less than tender loving care, but as you enter your thirties and forties, you just can't get away with it anymore. The more unconscious a woman is of her harmful diet and lifestyle choices, the more likely she is to have a difficult time with premenopause syndrome. Simply giving yourself the luxury of your own attention—what makes you sick, what makes you well—empowers you to make positive choices. And that is healing all by itself.

Chapter 15

❖

How Exercise Affects Your Hormone Balance

A century ago, women didn't have to think much about "getting their exercise." The keeping of a house, preparing of meals, and upbringing of children kept them on their feet, walking, lifting, digging, and reaching from morning to night. What would we do without our ready-made supermarket meals, department store clothing, and time-saving kitchen gadgets? How much time would you have to devote to something sedentary like watching TV if you had to cultivate and prepare enough food to feed your family, sew your own garments, and raise and slaughter your own livestock? One thing's for sure, you wouldn't need to invest in expensive exercise gadgets to stay fit. You would be using your body as it was intended to be used, keeping muscles and bones strong and joints supple with constant use.

Modern conveniences have since freed us from physical labor almost entirely, but there has been a price to pay for this freedom. It's as though the time saved with modern conveniences has been filled twice over with other duties, other obligations, and other necessities of life that require us to sit still for hours on end in cars and chairs.

Over the past couple of decades, lack of exercise has become a major public health issue. Study after study has shown that if you don't exercise regularly, you are at an exponentially higher risk of most diseases, including heart disease and breast cancer. Not only are you less likely to die young if you exercise regularly, but you are more likely to get greater enjoyment out of the years you do live.

Industrialized nations have become sedentary. According to the 1996 American Surgeon General's Report on Physical Activity and Health, 60 percent of Americans don't exercise regularly. Of that 60 percent, 25 don't exercise at all. Cars do laps around parking lots just to get a spot nearer to the door. Most people wouldn't dream of walking a mile to run an errand. An unprecedented number of children spend more time sitting in front of the TV than they spend playing outside. Many adults think of exercise as some kind of punishment for overindulgence, a sort of penance that will no longer be due once we've shed those few extra pounds we've been meaning to lose.

In many cultures, practices that harmonize mind with

body, like yoga and tai chi, are part of peoples' lives from childhood on. In Western cultures, however, priority hasn't been placed on this kind of self-care. A premium is not placed on health and well-being but rather on achievement and material wealth.

When we do make an effort to get fit, we are often swept off track by the various schools of thought on the subject. Bombardment by advertising, infomercials, and books by well-meaning professionals is enough to make you shrug your shoulders and go back to the couch.

If you haven't yet been able to get going with an exercise program, now is the ideal time. There are a lot of other shifts happening in your life as you regain balance: dietary changes, using natural hormones and supplements, and being more aware of how all your choices affect your health. Just taking a walk around the block every day is a big step in the right direction, as is the simple awareness that it's good to move—bending, reaching, stretching, lifting, pulling, and pushing. Although we're not necessarily advocates of a strict exercise regimen in the gym, if you choose to go that route there are some guidelines that will help you get the most out of your time and energy that also apply to other types of exercise.

The ideal exercise program includes cardiovascular (aerobic) exercise, strength exercises, and stretching. There is a virtually infinite number of ways to incorporate these three kinds of exercise into your life in a way that is pleasurable so that exercise can become another tool for staying on an even keel.

Without regular exercise, we become unable to deal

with even the slightest physical stress, and our bones deteriorate. After years of inactivity, we throw our backs lifting a bag of groceries and pull muscles just trying to get out of the car. We lose our sense of balance and depth perception. When we don't maintain our physical selves, we begin to feel unconnected to our bodies, causing us to ignore early warning pain and illness signals. The good news is that the musculoskeletal, neuroendocrine, and cardiovascular systems are quick to adapt themselves as soon as we start to exercise, and *everyone* can build muscle and improve stamina and balance once they get moving.

The concept of balance applies as much or more to exercise as it does to every other facet of life. Exercising too hard lowers your immune defenses and your antioxidant levels, but moderate exercise has the opposite effect. The idea here is to nurture and care for your body, not to beat up on it. If you are extremely fatigued after exercise, back off and pay more attention to balancing your hormones and diet for a while. Trying to force yourself to exercise through fatigue is counterproductive. On the other hand, moderate exercise after a stressful day at the office can be very soothing. As always, explore your options and find what works best for you.

We all know exercising is good for our health. But do you know what improves as you move your body? Here are some of the benefits you can expect:

• Your heart and blood vessels are strengthened, so they can keep blood circulating throughout the body without as much effort. New capillaries (microscopic blood vessels) form throughout the body, further improving circulation.

- Your muscles become hardier and develop greater endurance, so everyday tasks feel easier and workouts feel exhilarating.
- Your bones and connective tissues are strengthened by weight-bearing and strength-training exercise. The younger you start to exercise, the more dense your bones become, and that means far less risk of osteoporosis in old age.
- Your risk of heart disease, high blood pressure, diabetes, breast cancer, and stroke all decrease dramatically.
- Your respiratory muscles are strengthened, allowing deeper and easier breathing during exercise and throughout the day.
- Exercise sweeps excess cortisol (stress hormones) from the bloodstream. That's why a good workout feels so soothing after a stressful day.
- Immunity is boosted after each exercise session, so a regular exercise program means better resistance against infectious diseases.
- Exercise causes an increase in the body's natural antioxidant defenses.
- High-density lipoprotein or HDL ("good") cholesterol is boosted by exercise.
- Sleep quality improves on days you work out.
- Women who exercise have more satisfying sex lives.

- When you exercise, your body makes hormones called endorphins, which are natural painkillers and mood enhancers.
- Exercise is a natural appetite suppressant and a good way to ease cravings.
- Menstrual cramps and PMS are soothed by a good workout.
- Increased muscle mass from strength training raises your body's energy requirements. That means more calories are expended all day long, every day. The idea that fat turns to muscle isn't true, but if you have more muscle, you burn more fat.
- If you exercise and eat according to our guidelines, you can expect to lose a few pounds. Excess body fat is a source of excess estrogen. Fat loss means lower estrogen levels, and for many women, this is an important step toward creating balance after years of estrogen dominance.

❖ AEROBICS 101

You don't have to go to an aerobics class to get aerobic exercise. Anything that gets the major muscle groups moving, your heart pumping harder, and your breaths coming faster is aerobic. Walking, running, cycling, swimming, and aerobic dancing all fall into this category. So do vacuuming the house and running around after a toddler in the park.

Exercise is the most natural thing in the world. Our bodies want to be moved and stretched on a regular basis.

In the days before treadmills, people had to do physical work all day long, so they paced themselves. Because we spend most of our days sitting, it's necessary to work out at a higher intensity to get the same benefits we could get from just being moderately active all day long. Because of our mostly sedentary lifestyles, we have to give the body a stronger exercise stimulus to cause the adaptations that support our health.

If you understand the concepts of frequency, intensity, and duration, you'll know everything you need to know to design your own aerobic exercise program. Frequency refers to the number of workouts per week. It's best to get at least three workouts, spaced through the week, though daily is ideal.

Intensity refers to how hard you work, that is, how much your heart rate increases (see the next section for guidelines) or how quickly you burn calories. If you walk for a half hour at three miles per hour, you can expect to expend 120 calories; if you walk for the same amount of time at four miles per hour, you'll burn closer to 165 calories. You'll always burn more calories during weight-bearing exercise if you are heavier; the more you weigh, the more calories you burn. Caloric expenditure also increases when you do hills. For every 3 percent grade, your body uses as much energy as it would take to go a mile per hour faster. The other thing to know about intensity is that the harder you work during your aerobic workout, the longer the "afterburn," the length of time after exercise that your body continues to use more energy than it does at rest.

Duration refers to the length of each workout. The minimum to aim for is twenty minutes, although in the case of exercise something is always better than nothing. If you only have ten minutes, take a walk anyway.

Consider all three of these factors when deciding on your aerobic exercise program. If you can only find time for three aerobic workouts a week, you can make them longer and a little more intense than if you do one every day. If you have an hour to exercise four times a week, you can go slower than if you only have twenty minutes on those four days.

✤ TAKE A WALK

Lace on a pair of comfortable shoes, put on a hat, and head out the door. Bring a watch and promise yourself you'll walk for ten minutes one way and ten minutes back. Walk as briskly as you can, spine tall, legs reaching forward long and pushing off behind, arms swinging freely. Try to walk in an area where there is little or no traffic—car exhaust can ruin an otherwise pleasant walk—and choose terrain suited to your fitness level. If you are in decent shape, choose a route with a few hills or sets of steps. If you're just starting out, you might want to go to a shopping center or indoor mall, where you know you won't have to climb any hills.

A good walk will make you feel just a little bit out of breath, and will make your heart beat about twice as fast as it does at rest. To measure your resting heart rate (RHR), take your pulse first thing in the morning, when you haven't woken to the alarm. Count it for a full minute. Most people will count between 65 and 90 beats. Record this number and check it again after a couple of months of regular exercise; it will probably be a few beats less. As you get in shape, your heart pumps more blood with each beat, and has to beat fewer times per minute to perfuse all the tissues throughout your body.

Here's a simple formula to calculate a target rate for your heart rate when you walk briskly.

1. Subtract your age from 220. This result is your age-predicted maximum heart rate (MHR).
2. Multiply your MHR by 65 percent (.65). This is the bottom number of beats (per minute) of your ideal heart rate range, or 65 percent of MHR.
3. Multiply your MHR by 85 percent (.85). This is the top number of beats (per minute) of your ideal heart rate range during exercise, or 85 percent of MHR.
4. Divide both numbers by six. When you take your pulse for ten seconds, you should fall between the two numbers from steps two and three.

On your walk, take your pulse at the turnaround point, counting the number of beats in ten seconds. If it's below your target range, better find a tougher route or pick up the pace!

Keeping track of heart rate is a good way to know when it's time to change your workouts. Once you've done the same one for a while, your cardiovascular system adapts to it and your heart rate won't go up quite as much. Then you'll know it's time to challenge yourself with a new route.

Find time for a walk every day if you can. Five walks a week is a good goal, or mix it up with other kinds of aerobic exercise: swimming, cycling, or dance exercise classes. Some women find it easier to keep exercising if they vary their routine, never doing the same thing two days in a row. Others like to get settled into a consistent daily program where they do the same thing each day. There's no right or wrong here, as long as you get moving and stay moving!

If you live in the inner city or in a part of the country that has an unforgiving climate, you may want to join a gym or invest in equipment to use in your home. Good gyms have knowledgeable, available staff to answer questions; plenty of equipment kept in good working order at all times; and clean facilities. Most gyms offer full class schedules of aerobic dance, stretching, strength training, and even yoga. There are more and more women-only gyms opening up to cater to women who feel self-conscious or intimidated in co-ed gyms.

If you'd rather get your workout at home, you might want to invest in a treadmill. Look for the kind with an electronic belt (not the kind you push with your feet) and an incline setting so that you can walk hills right in your own living room while you watch the news. Treadmills are better than stationary bikes because you get aerobic exercise plus the impact of weight-bearing exercise which is good for your bones.

❧ STRENGTH TRAINING

Your muscles, bones, and cardiovascular system respond specifically to the amount of physical stress placed upon them. In sedentary people, bones and muscles lose mass rapidly. The economy of the body construes the lack of activity as a sign that those tissues don't need to be strong. Physical activity stimulates the body to lay down proteins (in muscle) and minerals and collagen (in bones). Staying active protects you from injuring yourself during day-to-day activities. It's almost as though you're tricking the body into maintaining muscle and bone that aren't really needed in our everyday lives.

Osteoporosis isn't a disease that comes on in old age. It starts in women who are still in the prime of their lives and creeps along very slowly as small amounts of mineral are lost from bone each day. Only after years and years of this slow attrition do bones become noticeably brittle. Resistance training, weight-bearing cardiovascular exercise like walking or jogging, natural progesterone, and a health-supporting diet are your best defenses against osteoporosis.

Resistance exercise includes weight lifting with machines or free weights, exercises with rubber tubing, and exercises where you use your own body weight for resistance, such as push-ups or squats. It also includes washing windows, polishing furniture, pushing a vacuum, scrubbing the floor, and lifting children, as well as hitting a tennis ball, swimming, and horseback riding (in the lower body). Hatha yoga incorporates poses supported by the strength of the muscles and can be considered a form of resistance training.

If you have a gym membership and weight lifting appeals to you, inquire about a personal training session to get one-on-one instruction on how to use the weight machines and free weights. Those who have never used weights may need more than one session to feel comfortable, and you'll want to have a session every month or two to update your program as you build your strength.

If you're working out at home, you'll want to get some dumbbells. A set of two five-pounders, two eight-pounders, and two twelve-pounders should be plenty to get you started. You can hire a trainer to come to your house to show you how to use your free weights, or start with a class at your local gym or Y.

It's a good idea to get at least two strength-training workouts a week, and it's ideal if you can find time for three. When you strength-train properly, you work just hard enough to break some of the microscopic fibers that make up the body of the muscle. Soreness after a good strength-training session is due to these microtears. The body fixes the damage, making the fibers a little sturdier in the process so that they won't break the next time they're stressed in this way. Over a period of three or four weeks your muscles have adapted to the new stresses you've placed on them, and you're ready to lift a little more weight. Don't do resistance training two days in a row because your muscles need at least a day between workouts to lay down new proteins where muscle fibers have been damaged.

The amount of weight you lift should be enough to exhaust the muscle group being used within one set of ten to twelve repetitions. Each repetition should be performed in a controlled, slow manner, without holding your breath. You can start out with one set per exercise, and gradually work your way up to three sets with at least thirty seconds of rest in between. If you want to split up your weight workouts, you can do some of your exercises one day and the rest on the following day so that you don't do any one exercise two days in a row.

❖ THE IMPORTANCE OF STRETCHING

Stretching should be an integral part of every aerobic or strength-training exercise you do. In fact, if you do nothing else in the way of exercise in any given day, at least do some stretching.

Even the most fanatical exercisers often skip stretching after workouts. It takes time and focus, and sometimes it hurts. The rewards are less tangible than those of aerobic and strength training. Don't give up on it, though. Stretching is your most important tool in the prevention of injury and is especially necessary for the health of your spine and the muscles that support it.

You don't have to wrap your legs around your neck or perform pretzel-shaped yoga poses to gain the benefits of stretching. It's about reaching your limits, at whatever level you're at right now, and gently pushing those limits.

Yoga is an excellent way to learn how to do beneficial stretching. You can buy a yoga video that emphasizes stretching, or you can take a class.

Don't stretch muscles that are cold and tight. The best time to stretch is after a workout, or at least after a five-minute warm-up to get your muscles and joints more supple. Ease into stretches rather than jerking or bouncing into them. A muscle suddenly stretched beyond its usual range of motion contracts reflexively to protect itself. Not only is this counterproductive when you're trying to stretch, it can also lead to muscle and tendon injury.

Once you've gotten to the point in a stretch where the pulling feels a little uncomfortable, you're at your limit. Hold the stretch there and breathe deeply, letting the muscles you're stretching relax further with each exhalation. You'll be surprised at how far your limit can move when you work this way. Hold each stretch for at least a minute.

Especially important areas to stretch are your lower back, your hamstrings (the muscles that run vertically up the back of the thigh), and your quadricep/hip flexor muscles (those that run from the knees to the pelvis). Keeping those areas limber allows your pelvis to stay in a neutral position rather than being tugged out of alignment by tight muscles and ligaments, which will help you avoid low back problems.

The following are some basic stretches for these key areas:

1. *Low back stretch.* Lie on your back and bring one knee into the chest, hugging it in with both arms and bringing your nose up to meet it. Hold for a few breaths, then switch legs. Repeat several times.

2. *Hamstring stretch.* Sit with your legs extended together in front of you, knees straight. Feel your weight resting on the two points of bone at the base of your pelvis. Take a deep breath in and extend your torso out over your legs, bending at the crease in the hip joint (not by rounding the lower back). Grasp your legs wherever you can reach them—feet, ankles, knees, or thighs—and try to keep your back flat. Extend your torso further on each inhalation and relax it toward your legs on each exhalation. If you're extremely tight, you can lie on your back and extend your legs up a wall to stretch the hamstrings.

3. *Quadricep/hip flexor stretch.* Stand up and take a large step forward with the left leg, landing in a lunge position. The left knee should be bent at a right angle, with the heel planted firmly, and the right knee and front of the right calf should be resting on the floor. The hands can be placed on either side of the left foot or the left thigh. Tuck your hips under you and with each exhalation, let the right hip sink toward the floor, sliding the right knee back if necessary. Hold for a minute, then switch sides.

❧ SUPPORTED POSES FOR RELAXATION

At the very end of a workout, or any time you please, you can use various poses to rejuvenate yourself. Yoga classes end with a pose called *chavasana*, which translates as "corpse pose." Being still for five or ten minutes does wonders for bringing the body and mind back to equilibrium. Try experimenting with the following poses.

1. *Embryo pose.* Come onto all fours and sit back on your heels, resting your forehead on the floor. You can either extend your arms over your head or reach back and clasp the sides of your feet. It's usually more comfortable to spread the knees and keep the feet touching, allowing your belly to sink down between your thighs. As you breathe, feel your back growing broader with each inhalation and a deepening relaxation as you exhale.

2. *Gentle backbend.* Pile up a few pillows or cushions and lie back over them. It should be a high enough pile to allow your head to hang toward the floor without touching it, with your hips on the floor. Relax your neck and face, feeling the head hang more heavily with each exhalation. Extend your arms over your head or to the sides, allowing the chest to open. (You can have your legs in a cross-legged position, extend them straight out, or place the soles of your feet together and let your knees open to the sides for a deep groin stretch.) To come out of this stretch, roll to one

side and use your hands to press yourself to a seated position.

3. *Spinal twist.* Lie on your back with arms spread at shoulder level, palms down, knees bent, feet on the floor. Let your knees fall to the right, keeping both shoulders on the floor, and turn your head to look toward the left hand. Relax and breathe deeply for a minute, then switch sides.

4. *Corpse pose.* Lie on your back with arms spread, palms up, and legs extended out comfortably. If you like, you can put a pillow under your legs or your neck—whatever feels most comfortable. Close your eyes and let yourself drift into a state of deep relaxation. Soothing music will help you let go and will also give you a sense of how long you've been there. You might try this pose for the length of a favorite song.

❖ YOUR BODY LOVES MOVEMENT

Always keep in mind that with exercise, something is always better than nothing. Adding any type of additional physical activity into a sedentary life makes a big difference. The benefits of accruing just thirty minutes of movement a day, even if it's not continuous, are enormous. The more you're able to do, the more benefit you'll experience.

Chapter 16

❖

How to Use Natural Progesterone

Now that you have a good idea of how to maintain and support your hormone balance through nutrition and exercise, this chapter will give you detailed guidelines for how to use natural progesterone and other natural hormones if you need to. By the time you finish this chapter you'll have a good understanding of why transdermal creams are far superior to any other way of administering progesterone. You'll understand why most commonly used blood tests that measure progesterone levels don't measure increases that occur with transdermal progesterone. And we'll address the specific needs of women who have their ovaries; women who have had total or partial hysterectomies; women who have endometriosis, fibroids, menstrual migraines, or PMS; and women using estrogen for irregular periods.

❖ WHY TRANSDERMAL CREAMS WORK THE BEST

Both estrogen and progesterone are wrapped in protein "coats" when they are released into the bloodstream from the ovaries. Estrogen is bound to sex hormone–binding globulin (SHBG) and progesterone is bound to cortisol-binding globulin (CBG). Fat-soluble, nonprotein-bound hormones do not mix well with the watery blood serum or plasma, so they get carried in the blood by "hitchhiking" on red blood cell membranes. When protein-bound, they are water-soluble. Only 2 to 10 percent of the progesterone in blood plasma is unbound and readily available for use. Less than 10 percent of the protein-bound hormone is active.

Transdermal progesterone, which means progesterone that is applied to the skin, passes through skin and into the layer of fat that lies beneath the skin, known as subcutaneous fat. The more progesterone deficient a woman is, the more readily it's absorbed. Although transdermal progesterone given to a progesterone-deficient woman shows up right away in a saliva hormone test, it can take as much as three months to show up as higher levels in blood tests. This gradual release achieved by transdermal progesterone is the only dosing method that approximates the natural physiologic release of the hormone from the ovaries.

The most compelling evidence that transdermal progesterone is indeed absorbed and distributed throughout the body is the relief of symptoms of estrogen dominance. Dr. Lee has seen breast fibrocysts disappear in only three or four menstrual cycles. The 1995 study conducted by K. J. Chang and associates, in which women used various combinations of hormone creams before breast surgery, showed that breast tissue levels of progesterone increased one hundred times, and estrogen-induced stimulation of breast cell proliferation (the first step toward breast cancer growth) is significantly inhibited, after just eight to ten days of using transdermal progesterone.

There are many problems with the use of oral progesterone. When you swallow a progesterone pill, it's broken down and absorbed through the intestinal wall, passing into the portal vein system. This carries the progesterone into the liver, where it's metabolized and excreted in bile. This is known as the first pass loss through the liver.

If a large enough dose is given—100 to 400 mg per day is the usual range for oral progesterone, as opposed to 15 to 30 mg per day for transdermal—the hormone surge exceeds the rate at which the liver can excrete it, so some of the breakdown products of progesterone metabolism pass into the blood plasma. Only about 10 percent of the oral dose ends up circulating as real progesterone. Whatever kind of progesterone is used, it is eventually broken down into these metabolites so that it can be flushed from the body.

Pregnanediones, pregnanolones, and pregnanediols are the major metabolites of progesterone. These substances don't function like true progesterone, and they compete for progesterone receptor sites. When physiologic doses of natural progesterone are used, the liver can keep up with excretion of these metabolites easily, but with the large doses used in oral progesterone, it can't get rid of them fast enough. Alterations in cell membranes and estrogen receptors result when progesterone metabolites are allowed to accumulate in the body. Especially noteworthy is that high doses of some of these substances affect neurotransmitter systems in the brain, impairing memory and causing lassitude and depression.

Large oral doses also result in a surge of progesterone that peaks in one or two hours, followed by a rapid decline and low levels for the rest of the day. Sublingual drops and vaginal suppositories of progesterone peak even more rapidly. Absorption through mucous membranes such as are found in the mouth and the vagina is extremely fast, and blood levels shoot up within twenty minutes. By the time ninety minutes have passed, levels have dipped way down again. This is not a physiologic way to give this hormone. The only reason to give progesterone this way is to prevent premenstrual migraines.

Transdermal progesterone maintains stable saliva levels for eight hours or more after application, so two small doses daily, providing a total of 15 to 20 mg per day, maintain levels throughout a 24-hour period.

❧ HORMONE LEVEL TESTING

Protein-bound progesterone is more soluble in the watery component of the blood. While protein-bound, only a small percentage of the hormone is active. This is also true of estrogens, testosterone, and the cortico-steroids. For this reason, blood serum concentration of these hormones is not an accurate measure of the amount of active hormone in the body because it misses the larger amount that is riding on red blood cell membranes.

Blood tests measure protein-bound hormone. Trans-dermally absorbed progesterone is not protein-bound but is most certainly biologically active. It's riding around in the bloodstream on red blood cell membranes and other fat-soluble constituents of the blood. Measuring endogenous (made in the body) hormone with blood testing is fairly accurate, but it simply isn't a reliable measure of progesterone levels when transdermal supplementation is being used. A far better test for bioavailable progesterone (and other steroid hormones) is by saliva assay.

Here's a typical situation for a woman starting on transdermal progesterone: She'll report to her physician that she's using it, and he or she will perform a blood test to check her levels. When the physician finds that levels are low, the conclusion is either that the cream doesn't have progesterone in it or that progesterone isn't absorbed through the skin.

If you use a cream that contains real natural progesterone, the first conclusion is incorrect, and the second conclusion is patently false. If you find yourself in this situation, you can take the opportunity to explain the saliva hormone radioimmunoassay (RIA) to your doctor. There are mucins in saliva in which nonprotein-bound (i.e., free) progesterone is soluble. Only the biologically active, unbound hormone shows up there, making the saliva RIA the most accurate, relevant, and convenient way to measure transdermal, free progesterone levels. The World Health Organization (WHO) has been using the saliva assay with good results for over five years. When saliva tests are used, increased levels are seen within three or four hours of using progesterone cream, maintained for three or four hours, and then drop gradually over three or four hours.

Normal levels of endogenous (made in the body) progesterone are about 12 to 24 ng/ml when measured by blood testing during the luteal phase or middle of the menstrual cycle when the corpus luteum is releasing progesterone.

When measured by salivary testing, the range you want is about 0.3 to 0.5 ng/ml, with 2 ng/ml at the upper limit. There's usually no reason to try to exceed this range, because this is as high as endogenous (produced by the body) progesterone production gets. However, excessive cortisol can blockade progesterone receptors, making them less able to respond to progesterone. High cortisol production occurs with stress of any kind, including emotional stress, trauma, and inflammation. Inflammatory bowel disease, for example, can induce high levels of cortisol and lead to significant reduction of progesterone effect and to estrogen dominance.

If serum or saliva tests indicate high estradiol levels, effort should be taken to reduce them. Estrogen levels can be lowered by preventing excess calorie intake, avoiding sugars and refined carbohydrates, maintaining a high-fiber diet, and supplementing with high-fiber products such as psyllium or rice bran. Excretion of estrogen is accomplished by the liver. It is important, therefore, to find a nutritionally oriented health care professional to prescribe nutrients that support the liver in this process.

❧ FINDING THE RIGHT DOSE OF NATURAL PROGESTERONE

People differ in almost every aspect of their physiology. We're not all built the same, and there's wide variation in physiologic and metabolic processes from person to person. It's not rational to order the same dose of any given medicine for everybody, and the same is true of natural progesterone.

Although medical professionals can give you guidelines to work within, it's up to you to find the best dose for your body. Ideally, you should be able to find the minimum amount you can use to gain and sustain relief from your symptoms. Because the safety of natural progesterone is so great, it's harmless to use a little more than you strictly need. That gives you plenty of room for experimentation.

All the dosage recommendations in this chapter are based on using a two-ounce container of progesterone cream that contains a total of 960 mg of progesterone. This amounts to 40 mg per ½ teaspoon, 20 mg per ¼ teaspoon, and 10 mg per ⅛ teaspoon.

Another way of looking at it is this: If one-third to one-half the container is used per month, over a 12- to 18-day time period, it means the dose is about 15 to 30 mg per day. This amounts to about ⅛ to ½ teaspoon per day for 12 to 18 days. This is the basic dose to use once you have attained balance. (This is not to say that other amounts of progesterone in a cream are wrong, but you need to adjust your dosage accordingly.) Dr. Lee doesn't recommend the superhigh dosage creams that contain 3,000 mg or more progesterone per two ounces because it's too easy to get too much, and we are striving for balance. *Please* avoid the "more is better" mentality when it comes to using progesterone cream. You have read over and over again in this book how important balance is, and if you use too much progesterone, you will create hormonal imbalance. If you are taking a physiologic dose (an amount approximating what your body would make itself under normal circumstances) and your symptoms don't go away after four to six months, or if they return, it's best to work in partnership with a competent health care professional to find out why.

At the recommended dosage, a progesterone-deficient woman who starts using the cream will find that in three to four months the progesterone in her body fat will reach physiologic equilibrium and the amount in the saliva will be consistent with what would be produced normally during an ovulatory cycle.

Dr. Lee tends to rely on relief of symptoms when figuring out the ideal dose for each woman. The right dose is the dose that works. (Question: How much water does it take to put out a fire? Answer: Enough.)

In a premenopausal woman (who is not preparing her uterus for pregnancy), about one-half of a two-ounce container used up in 24 to 25 days, or about ¼ teaspoon per day, will restore good physiologic levels of progesterone in one to two months. After that, one-third of a container (closer to ⅛ teaspoon per day) will maintain these levels. Women who are closer to actual menopause may need higher doses.

It's up to you to figure out just how to achieve your monthly dosing goal. The cream can be applied once or twice a day. Dr. Lee advises a divided dose, with a larger dose at bedtime and a smaller dose in the morning. Getting each dab of cream to be exactly the right size isn't that important here, because there's a buffering effect as the progesterone is absorbed into subcutaneous fat. The release of the hormone into the bloodstream stays relatively steady even if daily doses vary a little.

Here are some general guidelines on how to get the most out of your progesterone cream dose.

- The larger the area of skin the dose is spread on, the greater the absorption.
- Sufficient time should be allowed for maximum absorption, which is one reason to apply the cream at bedtime.
- Apply the cream to thinner and less keratinized skin with high capillary density—places where you blush. Biochemist David Zava has found that the best spots

are the palms (if they aren't calloused), chest, inner arms, neck, and face. The soles of the feet are also good if they're not thickened from walking barefoot. Contrary to what was advised in Dr. Lee's first book, we now know that the skin of the buttocks, inner thighs, and low abdomen are not quite as good.

- Other ingredients in the cream or in other skin applications can impede absorption. Use only reputable creams (see a list of options on page 392) and don't apply other skin creams in areas where you apply natural progesterone.

- Another reason to use the cream at bedtime is that it can be calming and help you sleep. If you want to apply it twice a day, use a larger dab at night and a smaller one in the morning.

- Since other ingredients of the cream may not be absorbed, continual use of any single skin area will eventually saturate that area, and this might reduce progesterone absorption. Rotate among three or four different skin sites on different days.

- Take at least three to seven days off every month. (Women who experience a severe recurrence of symptoms during the break can take as little as three days off. Otherwise it's best to give it a week.) This break protects against endometrial thickening in the uterus by allowing for complete shedding of the uterine lining each month—a menstrual period. In premenopausal women, progesterone deficiency causes a "tuning-down" of estrogen receptors; when women begin using progesterone cream, this reactivates those receptors. This can temporarily cause buildup of the endometrium, with spotting and irregular bleeding. Most women find that the estrogenic symptoms disappear within a couple of cycles.

Guidelines for Premenopausal Women Who Are Menstruating but Not Ovulating

Salivary assays done during the luteal or midcycle when progesterone levels would normally be at their highest can determine whether you're having anovulatory cycles. If your progesterone levels are low, that indicates that you haven't ovulated. If you have estrogen-dominance symptoms, that's also a pretty good indicator that you're not ovulating. Your health care professional can help you determine where you fall.

In one study of a group of 18 regularly cycling women, with an average age of twenty-nine, 7 of them (39 percent) were found to be anovulatory and were not producing progesterone during the luteal phase. A lot of women who appear normal for their age group are actually not ovulating and have very low progesterone levels.

If this is you, over the course of a month use ¼ to ½ of a two-ounce container of cream that contains approximately 960 mg per container (240 to 480 mg per month). Your goal is to approximate the 15 to 24 mg per day that an ovulating woman makes during the second half of her cycle. The length of this cycle can vary from 12 to 18 days, depending on how early in your cycle you ovulate and how long your cycle is. Women's sensitivity to hormones differs tremendously, so your dose will depend on your individual sensitivity.

Begin your first month of progesterone cream use between days 10 and 12 of your menstrual cycle, counting the first day of your period as day 1. Continue until the last day before your expected period, which for most women is between 26 and 30 days. (If you don't know how long your cycle is because you have had irregular bleeding, or if your cycles have been very short or very long, use your intuition and pick a day.) If your period starts before your chosen last day, stop using the cream and begin counting again to day 10, 11, or 12.

If you can feel it when you ovulate, or if you can tell by changes in your vaginal mucus that you have ovulated, you don't need to use the cream that month. (It's also okay to use the progesterone cream if you have ovulated.) If you have had irregular cycles, it may take up to three months to begin having a more normal menstrual cycle.

It's best to synchronize your natural progesterone supplementation with your body's own hormonal cycles as much as possible. Menstrual dysfunction is usually the result of more than just progesterone deficiency. Factors such as stress, diet, and cortisol production play important roles in this matter. The cooperation between the hypothalamus (the part of the brain that controls the endocrine system), the pituitary gland (the "master gland" that sends out instructions to other glands throughout the body), and ovaries may be out of sync because the body is out of balance. Adding progesterone at the right times in the right amounts helps this complex system regain its equilibrium.

Ovulation often begins to be irregular eight to ten years before actual menopause. Each anovulatory cycle sends a woman deeper into estrogen dominance as body-fat progesterone stores are depleted. Very thin women with little body fat go into estrogen dominance much more quickly. The first one or two months of transdermal progesterone is used to replenish body-fat stores, so it makes sense to use higher doses during that time. If you are having outright symptoms of estrogen dominance, use a full container (960 mg or 40 to 50 mg per day) for three weeks out of the month for a few months, and then cut it down to 12 to 18 days.

We can't emphasize enough that the bottom line in progesterone dosing is always observed physiologic effects. Are your PMS symptoms improved? Are you gaining less weight before your periods? Are your breast or uterine fibrocysts getting smaller? Are your moods steadier? Are you less anxious? It's all about working to find the dose that corrects the problem, then reducing that dose to the minimum needed to maintain the desired effect.

In premenopausal women who have been progesterone deficient for years, it's common that the initial application of progesterone will cause water retention, headaches, and swollen breasts—symptoms of estrogen dominance. This happens because the estrogen receptors shut down by progesterone deficiency are "waking up."

It's important to remember that these symptoms will disappear in two weeks to two or three months.

Guidelines for Women with Endometriosis

When you have endometriosis you want to use progesterone cream from day 8 to day 26 of your cycle to reduce the effects of estrogen, which stimulates the endometrial growth, just taking a short week off to refresh your hormone receptors. Your ultimate goal is to find the least dose of progesterone necessary to control endometrial stimulation.

Use progesterone cream from day 8 to days 26 to 30 (pick the day that most closely approximates the end of your normal cycle) each month, using up to an ounce (480 mg) of cream per week, or about 68 mg daily, until just before menstruation. It will take up to six months for symptoms to be controlled, and even then they may not dissipate entirely. Once outbreaks of endometriosis are more tolerable, decrease the dose to as close to two ounces a month from day 12 to the end of your cycle as possible. Increase the dose again if it flares up.

If the high doses of progesterone cream make you sleepy, that's an indication that you're taking too much. Reduce the dose until the sleepiness goes away.

Guidelines for Women with Uterine Fibroids

With the exception of cancer or severe uterine bleeding, before you allow a surgeon to remove your uterus, it's worth trying the same program we recommend for women who are not ovulating—one ounce of cream used from days 10, 11, or 12 of your cycle, to days 26 to 30, or you can even start as early as day 8. Ultrasound tests can be obtained initially and after three months to check results. A good result would show the fibroid size had not increased or had decreased by 10 to 15 percent. If so, this treatment program can be continued until menopause, after which the reduced estrogen production allows lower doses of progesterone to be used. With postmenopausal estrogen levels, fibroids usually atrophy.

Guidelines for Women with Breast Fibrocysts

Breast fibrocysts are generally due to estrogen dominance and respond well to progesterone therapy. Progesterone cream at 15 to 20 mg per day from ovulation until the day or two before your period starts will usually result in a return to normal breast tissue in three to four months. You can also take 400 IU of vitamin E at bedtime every night, as well as 300 mg of magnesium and 50 mg of vitamin B6 a day. For many women it helps to cut out coffee and reduce sugar and fat. Once the fibrocysts are under control, taper off the natural progesterone to the minimum dose needed to maintain those results.

Guidelines for Women Using Estrogen Supplements

Some women who have irregular bleeding are prescribed estrogen by their doctors. This is a misguided approach. There's really no good reason to give estrogen to women who are still menstruating. Unless you're close to actual menopause and experiencing blatant estrogen-deficiency symptoms such as hot flashes, night sweats, and vaginal dryness, the very fact that you're menstruating indicates that you're very unlikely to be deficient in estrogen.

You can reduce your estrogen dose by half when you add progesterone, and gradually taper off the estrogen completely. If you are using estrogen tablets, simply cut them in half or take one every other day. If you are using a patch, you may want to try cutting out a dime-size, circular piece of tape that will cover half of the patch. Place the tape over the skin and put the patch over it. Some women who try this complain of skin irritation from the tape; if this happens, ask your doctor to switch you to oral estrogen while you decrease your dosage over time.

Guidelines for Specific Premenopause Problems

For women with PMS: PMS usually involves stress and higher levels of the hormone cortisol. Cortisol competes with progesterone for common receptors, so you may need a higher dose. For the first month or two, use up a full two ounces from days 10 to 12 to days 26 to 30. Dr. Lee advises women treating PMS to use the cream in a crescendo pattern, with small dabs at night starting on days 10 to 12 and gradually increasing to two dabs per day morning and night. Finish off the last three or four days with bigger dabs, using up whatever remains of your monthly goal (usually two ounces to start, sometimes tapering off to one once symptoms are relieved). Since PMS is a syndrome with multiple causative factors, it is wise to seek guidance in matters of stress management, diet, and other nutritional advice.

For women with menstrual migraine: Use natural progesterone during the ten days before your period (days 16 to 26, for example). When you feel the characteristic "aura" that usually precedes migraines, apply ¼ to ½ teaspoon of cream every three to four hours, until your symptoms cease (usually this happens in only one or two applications). Sublingual drops, which are in a base of vitamin E oil, may be more effective, because they are absorbed rapidly and cause a quick spike in progesterone levels. A sublingual dose of 40 to 50 mg should do the trick. You can also apply the cream directly to your neck or your temples.

Guidelines for Premenopausal Women Who Have Had a Hysterectomy or Ovariectomy

Complete hysterectomy, the nonmedical term that means removal of both the uterus and the ovaries, is also known as "surgical menopause," and its abruptness is hard on the body. If you have had your ovaries surgically removed, natural progesterone can help you bring your body back into balance.

For women without ovaries: Use 15 to 20 mg per day of progesterone for 25 days of the calendar month, with five to seven days without it. That should add up to about an ounce a month. For a month or two after surgery you may need to take up to 50 mg a day to restore balance.

If you are using estrogen replacement, when you begin

taking progesterone, immediately reduce your estrogen by half. You can either break the tablets in half or take one every other day. If you have been progesterone deficient, your estrogen receptors will up-regulate when you start using the progesterone, so the estrogens have a more intense effect. Water retention, headaches, and other symptoms of estrogen dominance can occur. You may want to use an entire two-ounce container of progesterone cream (40 to 50 mg per day) for the first one or two months to restore balance. When you're taking higher doses like this, it's best to take a higher dose (20 to 30 mg) at night and a smaller dose (10 to 20 mg) in the morning.

For women with ovaries but without a uterus: Follow the instructions above for "women who are menstruating but not ovulating." A hysterectomy significantly compromises blood supply to the ovaries, so their ability to produce progesterone is quite quickly reduced, and within two years estrogen production falls to post-menopausal levels.

For women using unopposed estrogen: As we've said elsewhere in this book, the conventional medical practice of putting women without a uterus on unopposed estrogen (without progesterone) is dangerous and misguided. You should *always* take progesterone along with estrogen. Since progesterone restores normal estrogen receptor sensitivity it is wise to reduce estrogen by 50 percent when you begin using progesterone. Further reductions of estrogen every two to three months will eventually lead to your "right" estrogen dose—which might be zero.

Chapter 17

—— ❧ ——

How to Use Other
Natural Hormones

*I*n addition to progesterone, there are other hormones that you can supplement as needed to achieve hormone balance. No hormone works in isolation. That's why we've placed such a strong emphasis on creating balance among them. This is accomplished through lifestyle changes and small physiologic doses of natural hormones that approximate what the body makes, rather than the use of large pharmacologic doses of synthetic hormones.

We've talked in great detail about progesterone and the estrogens, and it's our feeling that natural progesterone, with its wide array of healing properties, is as close to "magic bullet" status as anything gets.

Dr. Lee did not supplement hormones such as DHEA when he had a clinical practice, but Dr. Hanley uses them extensively and has created some guidelines you can follow.

The following hormones are produced in more than adequate amounts in most young people, but their production dwindles as we age, beginning as early as the mid-thirties. Poor diet, undue stress, and lack of self-care over the years accelerates this process, and it may be the reason we age faster and suffer from diseases like heart disease and cancer when we don't embrace a health-promoting lifestyle.

❖ ESTROGEN

For more details about estrogen, you can refer to chapter 3.

If estrogen is needed for symptoms such as hot flashes and vaginal dryness, find the lowest dose that controls symptoms. Use estrogen on the same days you use progesterone, leaving five to seven days without either hormone. Because women without ovaries continue to make estrogen in their body fat, and because natural progesterone makes estrogen receptors more sensitive, many find that they can stop estrogen completely after five or six months. As you reduce estrogen further, don't hesitate to ask your doctor for pills, patches, or a cream containing smaller doses.

Natural estrogens (for humans) are estrone, estradiol, and estriol. We've said it before and we'll say it again: Premarin is not natural unless you're half horse and half human. It's completely unnecessary for you to use it, and we don't recommend it.

There are creams available that contain both progesterone and estrogens, and there are creams that only contain one or more estrogens. Your doctor can have a compounding pharmacist make up a cream for you that contains the hormones you need in the amounts you need. All the available evidence we have so far indicates that estriol is the safest estrogen to use to control menopausal symptoms, and that it may even be protective against breast cancer. The jury is still out on whether estriol is as effective as the others in slowing bone loss.

The estrogens vary considerably both in their potency and their ability to be absorbed through the skin. Estradiol is extremely potent, having effects at minute doses, and it absorbs fairly well through the skin (transdermally). Estriol, on the other hand, requires double or triple the dose to achieve the same effects and is not well absorbed through the skin. Estrone falls in between. Thus, the estrogen creams that contain 80 percent estriol and smaller amounts of estradiol and estrone may actually be *delivering* nearly equal amounts of these estrogens relative to their potency in the body.

In general, the recommended doses for the estrogens are 1 to 4 mg daily for estriol, 0.25 to 0.5 mg daily for estradiol, and 0.3 to 0.625 mg daily for estrone. If the lowest doses work to alleviate your symptoms, or if you are having estrogen-dominance symptoms, then try taking them every other day or even every third day. In other words, you're looking for the smallest dose that will relieve your symptoms. If your only estrogen-deficiency symptom is vaginal dryness or atrophy, then you can apply an estriol cream vaginally a few times a week.

We can't emphasize strongly enough that no woman, with or without a uterus or ovaries, should ever take estrogen alone. It should *always* be combined with natural progesterone. There are no exceptions to this.

❧ DHEA

DHEA, or dehydroepiandrosterone, is a steroid hormone just like estrogens and progesterone. It's made in the adrenal glands, which make over 150 different hormones. Estrogens and testosterone are made from DHEA (or progesterone) throughout the body. The amount of DHEA made in our bodies is greater than any other of the adrenal steroid hormones. All but 5 percent of it is bound to sulfur molecules, making it more soluble in blood plasma and providing us with ample reserves to draw from. We know that DHEA is important for the maintenance of health, but an understanding of its specific actions has so far eluded researchers.

Between the ages of twenty and twenty-five, DHEA production peaks. Men produce more than women, but both sexes make about 2 percent less every year after the age of twenty-five. By the time a woman reaches her mid- to late forties, DHEA levels can be quite low.

The onset of diseases like cancer, heart disease, allergies, diabetes, and autoimmune diseases correlate with this gradual drop in DHEA levels. We don't know yet if this means that lower DHEA levels play a causal role in these diseases, or if lower DHEA levels are a biomarker for aging in the same sense that gray hair and bifocals are. We do know that in elderly people, higher levels of DHEA mean better health and longer life span. When people with low levels are given DHEA they experienced a significant boost in energy, immune function, ability to adapt to stress, feelings of well-being, and sex drive. Many feel that DHEA replacement actually takes years off their chronologic ages. There is also evidence that adequate DHEA levels help protect against osteoporosis.

If you are interested in DHEA and you're over forty, ask your doctor to do a blood test to measure your DHEAS (the sulfur-bound form) levels. This is a fairly accurate way to measure the amount of DHEA in your body, but you can also have salivary assays done for this hormone. The normal blood range for women between the ages of forty and fifty is 400 to 2,500 ng/ml; for women over fifty, it falls to 200 to 1,500 ng/ml. Those are pretty big ranges. If yours falls in or below the low half of the range, and you are generally fatigued and have worked to balance your other hormones, diet, and stress levels, you might want to give DHEA a try.

You can try using 5 to 10 mg a day. Don't buy products advertising themselves as "DHEA precursors," including wild yam creams and pills, because there's no guarantee your body can make the conversion.

One word of caution: DHEA can have masculinizing effects on women, and in excess it can have the opposite effect of the low dosages, increasing your risk of diabetes and heart disease. This is much more true of women than men. If you start to see changes like acne, hair loss, or the growth of facial hair, cut back to 5 mg every other day or stop taking it. These side effects are entirely reversible with decreased dosage or discontinuation of DHEA. Have your DHEAS levels checked periodically as long as you're using it.

✦ PREGNENOLONE

Pregnenolone is made from cholesterol by mitochondria and is the compound within cells from which DHEA, progesterone, estrogens, cortisol, and testosterone are created. It would seem that taking large doses of pregnenolone, which is very safe and has no hormone effect itself, would be a good way to reach hormone balance, giving the body what it needs to make its other steroid hormones. Unfortunately, it doesn't work that way. Pregnenolone supplementation doesn't raise concentrations of other steroid hormones.

Pregnenolone does appear to have some benefit on rheumatoid arthritis symptoms. Those who have this autoimmune disease can try 10 to 50 mg three times daily. Give it at least a month to work. Some clinicians use doses of 100 to 200 mg daily, but please, only use these amounts under the supervision of a health care professional who will monitor your health.

Researchers have recently discovered that pregnenolone blocks receptors for the neurotransmitter gamma-aminobutyric acid (GABA). High GABA levels can have the effect of blocking memory and pregnenolone seems to offset that effect. It also increases brain cell activity. Those who have problems learning or remembering may benefit from 50 to 100 mg of pregnenolone between meals, but again, at these doses, please work in partnership with a health care professional and monitor your hormone levels.

❧ THE CORTICOSTEROIDS

Corticosteroids are made by the adrenal cortex in response to long-term stress. They include cortisol, which is a glucocorticoid that regulates immune response, opposes insulin, and stimulates conversion of proteins to glucose in the liver (gluconeogenesis). Other corticosteroids such as corticosterone help regulate mineral balance. Aldosterone is the most potent of these, acting on the renal tubule (kidney) to promote retention of sodium and the increased excretion of potassium. You might also see these hormones referred to as cortisones, which has become a generic term for adrenal cortex hormones.

These hormones respond to any stressors that increase energy requirements. Fasting, infection, intense exercise, pain, or emotional stress stimulate the secretion of a releasing hormone from the hypothalamus in the brain, which tells the adrenals to secrete extra cortisol. There's also a regular daily cycle of cortisol release into the bloodstream, with peaks in the morning and late afternoon and lows in midafternoon and during deep sleep.

Cortisol is extremely important to survival when stress

of any sort is present. If an animal can be made stress-free, the lack of cortisol is not life-threatening. But without the corticosteroids, we couldn't survive even the slightest stress. People who have had their adrenal glands removed or whose adrenals don't make enough cortisol are in danger of death from even mild illness. These people must use cortisol replacement for the rest of their lives, increasing their dose at any sign of extra stress or infection.

Excessive cortisol, on the other hand, creates a broad range of undesirable side effects including truncal obesity, elevated blood glucose, hypertension, "moon" face, fatty accumulation (called a buffalo hump) behind the neck and upper thorax, osteoporosis, bruising, a susceptibility to fungal infections, and disorders of the immune system. If produced by excessive stimulation by pituitary adrenocorticotropic hormone (ACTH), the resulting disease is called Cushing's disease. If resulting from excessive adrenal production independent of pituitary control, the disease is called Cushing's syndrome.

Chronic stress leads to chronic high levels of cortisol in the bloodstream, which leads to a greater need for both DHEA and progesterone to maintain balance. In addition to the symptoms of Cushing's disease and syndrome, chronic excessive cortisol is toxic to brain cells in high concentrations. A lifetime of high cortisol levels may be a primary cause of Alzheimer's disease and senile dementia. High cortisol is also a primary cause of osteoporosis because it blocks the bone-building effects of progesterone.

The way this hormone is used in conventional medicine is another good example of the dramatic difference between physiologic and pharmacologic dosing with hormones. People who take powerful synthetic cortisone drugs like prednisone, prednisolone, and dexamethasone for their anti-inflammatory effects suffer side effects like swelling of the face, acne, unwanted hair growth on the face and body, lowered resistance to infection, weight gain around the midriff, menstrual irregularities, and psychological problems ranging from depression to anxiety to outright psychosis. With long-term use, these medications cause adrenal cortisol production to shut down completely, so stopping the drug can cause fatal complications. Natural hydrocortisone or cortisone acetate, used in small doses several times a day, has very little incidence of side effects and has been used successfully to treat symptoms of adrenal insufficiency.

Supplementing natural hydrocortisone or cortisone acetate in doses of 2.5 to 5 mg two to four times daily can be a safe and effective way to replenish depleted adrenals. (Too much taken later in the day can cause insomnia, so adjust your dosage accordingly, or don't take it later in the day.) Proper use of natural cortisols can correct problems as diverse as asthma, rheumatoid arthritis, and chronic fatigue. However, it's very important to combine the cortisone supplementation with lots of rest, good nutrition, and hormone balance, with the goal of healing the adrenal glands and not having to use it every day. Once you have brought your body back into balance you can use it occasionally as needed, which you'll know by your symptoms.

We suggest that you use natural cortisone supplementation with the guidance of a health professional, because even natural cortisone isn't safe if you take too much, and it's a delicate balance to maintain. If you take it when you don't really need it, it can cause problems. If your doctor doesn't know about William McK. Jefferies's ground-breaking book *Safe Uses of Cortisone*, inform him or her that it contains all the necessary information on how and when to prescribe physiologic amounts of natural cortisone.

If you don't have the symptoms of cortisol deficiency but are living an extremely hectic life, working and playing too hard and not taking time to get enough sleep and to relax, you're probably making too much cortisol. Even if your adrenals can sustain that kind of energy without ever running down, you're still at risk from chronically high cortisol levels. Optimal health is achieved with a balance of activity and rest.

❧ TESTOSTERONE

Women make about a tenth as much testosterone as their male counterparts. The adrenal glands are responsible for maintaining adequate testosterone levels in women.

As is the case with most other hormones and aging, female production of testosterone decreases with age. Studies of hormone replacement in women have shown that adding a low dose of (natural) testosterone can sometimes enhance the positive effects of other hormones. The other side of this coin is that in many cases, as the ovaries wind down, women show signs of becoming more androgen (male hormone) dominant rather than estrogen dominant, and testosterone will only exaggerate that process.

Facial hair and male-type pattern baldness are indicative of this shift. This can happen in premenopausal, estrogen-dominant women as well, because testosterone clearance from the body is partly controlled by the balance between estrogen and progesterone. Excess estrogen decreases testosterone clearance and natural progesterone enhances it. In estrogen-dominant women, testosterone hangs around in the body for a longer time, and the end result is as though more testosterone were being made. This is why progesterone cream tends to reverse the androgenic changes mentioned above.

If you have used progesterone cream for at least six months and still have a low libido, you might want to try a very small amount of some natural testosterone. It's easy to get it in a cream from a compounding pharmacist. The optimal dose is usually in the range of 0.5 to 2 mg in the morning. If you find you are getting androgenic symptoms, reduce the dose or stop taking it for a while.

Testosterone is available only by prescription. If you're interested, talk with your physician. Be sure to use only a natural form, as synthetics like methyltestosterone are powerful and can have unpleasant side effects.

A note about men and testosterone. As men age, progesterone levels fall, testosterone becomes converted to dihydrotestosterone (DHT), and estradiol levels rise. The effect of this is weight gain, some breast enlargement, an enlarged prostate gland, and, sometimes, prostate cancer. Testosterone actually protects against prostate cancer whereas DHT does not protect against the carcinogenic effects of increased estradiol. The conversion of testosterone to DHT is promoted by the enzyme 5α-reductase. The action of this enzyme is inhibited by progesterone (and saw palmetto extract). Thus, progesterone is not only the precursor of testosterone synthesis but also inhibits its conversion to DHT. This is important since testosterone antagonizes and limits estradiol effects, thus preventing prostate cancer. The importance of progesterone in protecting against prostate cancer is just now penetrating conventional medicine. This would appear to be a fruitful avenue for further research.

❖ ANDROSTENEDIONE

Androstenedione is a steroid hormone that is a precursor to testosterone and estrogens, and it can theoretically act as a DHEA precursor. Secreted from the adrenals and the ovaries into the circulation, it has its own jobs to do before being converted into other hormones in the liver. In older women it travels from the ovaries to the fat cells where it is converted to estrogen.

Androstenedione is a popular supplement for bodybuilders, who use it to boost their testosterone levels, increasing muscle mass and decreasing the length of time needed to recover from hard workouts. Many of the positive effects of supplemental testosterone, including enhanced energy, libido, and sense of well-being, have also been attributed to androstenedione. Androstenedione may also be involved in maintaining the strength of bones. It's converted to estradiol in the bones themselves, and estradiol helps slow bone loss.

If you have testosterone-deficiency symptoms but aren't ready to try testosterone, androstenedione just might do the trick. It's available in health food stores. Use very small doses, no more than 50 mg twice a week, to see if your energy, libido, and mood are improved. Again, this can be a powerfully androgenic, or male, hormone, or it can increase estrogen levels, so it should be used with great care. It's recommended that women not use both androstenedione and DHEA or testosterone.

Glossary

❖

amenorrhea	absence of menstruation
androgenic	producing masculine characteristics
anovulatory	suspension or cessation of ovulation
carcinogen	any cancer-producing substance
catalyst	any substance that enhances the rate or velocity of a chemical reaction
chromosome	a molecule that comprises the gene (genome), or hereditary factor, composed of DNA or RNA
conjugated	in biochemistry, one compound combined with another
corpus luteum	small yellow glandular mass in the ovary formed by an ovarian follicle after ovulation (release of its egg [ovum])
corticosteroid	hormone produced by the adrenal cortex
cytoplasm	the watery protoplasm of a cell,

	excluding the nucleus
diuretic	substance that increases urine production
DNA	deoxyribonucleic acid, the basic molecular subunit of chromosomes
dysmenorrhea	painful menstruation
endocrine	refers to organs (glands) that secrete hormones
endogenous	developing or originating within the body
endometrium	the inner lining of the uterus
enzyme	an organic compound, usually a protein, capable of facilitating a specific chemical reaction
exogenous	originating outside of the body
follicle	a very small sac or cavity composed of cells, e.g., the ovarian follicle that produces the ovum
gonadal	refers to the gamete-producing glands, i.e., ovaries and testes
gonadotropic	refers to hormones that affect or stimulate gonads
gram	unit of mass (weight); about one-twenty-eighth of an ounce
homeostasis	the body's ability to maintain a stable internal environment
hydroxylation	the addition of a hydroxyl radical (-OH) to a compound
hypermenorrhea	excessive bleeding with menses
hypothalamus	neural centers of the limbic brain

	just above the pituitary that control visceral activities, water balance, sleep, and hormone production by the pituitary
hysterectomy	surgical removal of the uterus
libido	sex drive
limbic brain	brain cortex below the corpus callosum and above the pituitary that contains neural centers controlling autonomic functions, homeostasis, and emotional sensation and responses, and regulates immune responses
luteinizing	refers to the maturation of ovarian follicles following ovulation, during which the follicle becomes the corpus luteum producing progesterone
mastodynia	painful breasts
metabolism	the biochemical process of living organisms by which substances are produced and energy is made available to the organism
microgram	one-millionth (10^{-6}) of a gram
milligram	one-thousandth (10^{-3}) of a gram
mineralcorticoid	an adrenal hormone that regulates sodium, potassium, and water balance
mitochondria	small organelles within the cytoplasm that are the site of

	converting sugar into energy
nanogram	one-billionth (10^{-9}) of a gram
oocyte	the cell that produces the ovum
oophorectomy	surgical removal of an ovary or ovaries
osteoblast	bone cell that forms new bone
osteoclast	bone cell that resorbs old bone
osteocyte	means bone cell; may become an osteoclast or an osteoblast
osteoid	the noncellular, collagenous matrix of bone
peptide	a class of low-molecular-weight compounds composed of several amino acids; a miniprotein
perimenopausal	referred to as premenopausal in this book—refers to the time preceding menopause when hormone changes are occurring
phyto-	denotes relationship to plants
premenopausal	prior to menopause, also called "perimenopausal"
resorption	the loss or dissolving away of a substance
serum	the watery, noncellular liquid of the blood
steroid	group name for compounds based on the cholesterol molecule, e.g., sex hormones and corticosteroids
sterol	compounds with a single hydroxyl group (-OH) soluble in fats, widely

	found in plants and animals. Cholesterol is a sterol.
synovial	referring to the inner lining of a joint
thermogenic	capable of inducing a rise in temperature
trans-	prefix referring to something altered from the natural state, such as transfatty acids
xeno-	combining form meaning strange or foreign

Resources

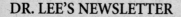

DR. LEE'S NEWSLETTER

The John R. Lee, M.D., Medical Letter. If you want to know what's on Dr. Lee's mind every month, this is the way to do it. Call (800) 528-0559, write to PO Box 84900, Phoenix, AZ 85071, or e-mail at info@john-leemd.com for more information.

SOURCES OF NATURAL PROGESTERONE CREAM

You can find progesterone creams in most health food stores these days, but many contain little to no real progesterone, so buyer beware. Regardless of the source, be sure you're getting the real thing. If the label says "wild yam extract" don't buy the product without confirming that it contains progesterone and not the so-called precursors such as diosgenin. KAL, Jason, and Country Life make progesterone creams that are widely available in health food stores.

Your doctor can order a progesterone cream from a compounding pharmacy, but be careful of the 10 percent creams that contain very high amounts of progesterone. Taking a higher-than-recommended dose does contribute to hormone balance. Dr. Lee recommends a 1.6 percent cream, with about 450-500 mg of progesterone per ounce with a 15 to 20 mg dose under most conditions.

Many natural progesterone creams contain ingredients other than progesterone that may be active, including "wild yam extract"—which is usually diosgenin—a variety of herbs, and aromatic oils. We do not know which are active and which aren't, or what biochemical effects these ingredients may or may not have, nor do we know what effect they may have when used by women who are pregnant or nursing. Dr. Lee does not recommend creams that contain DHEA unless you are working with a health care professional.

There are plenty of perfectly good progesterone creams that aren't on this list, many of them private label versions of these creams. Due to space limitations we can't list them all.

The following creams contain real progesterone in at least the amount recommended by Dr. Lee.

Dr. Lee does not endorse any one progesterone cream or company, nor does he make any money from the sale of any progesterone cream.

AIM International, Inc.
3904 E Flamingo Ave

Nampa, ID 83687
(208) 465-5116

Maker of Renewed Balance progesterone cream. (This cream contains a higher-than-recommended amount of progesterone.)

Broadmoore Labs Inc.
3875 Telegraph Rd 294
Ventura, CA 93003
(800) 822-3712

Maker of Natra-Gest and DermaGest progesterone creams.

Easy Way International
5340 Commerce Cir #E
Indianapolis, IN 46237
(800) 267-4522

Maker of Gentle Changes progesterone cream.

HM Enterprises
5215 Wexford Ln
Norcross, GA 30071
(800) 742-4773

Maker of Happy PMS and Adam's Equalizer progesterone creams.

The Health and Science Research Inst.
141 Glover Ln
Crawfordville, Fl 32327
(800) 222-1415; www.health-science.com

Maker of Serenity for Women progesterone cream.

International Health
8704 E Mulberry St
Scottsdale, AZ 85251
(602) 874-1419; outside Arizona: (800) 481-9987

Distributor of Ess-Pro 7 natural progesterone cream.

Karuna
42 Digital Dr., #7,
Novato, CA 94949 (800) 826-7225, (888) 749-8643
karunacorp@earthlink.net

Maker of PhytoGest cream.

Kenogen
P.O. Box 50423, Eugene, OR 97405, (541) 345-9855

Maker of Raymond Peat's progesterone in vitamin E oil.

Kokoro, LLC
PO Box 597
Tustin, CA 92781
(800) 599-9412; (714) 538-3635;
www.kokorohealth.com

Maker of Kokoro Balance cream.

Life-flo Health Care Products
8146 N 23rd Ave Ste E
Phoenix, AZ 85021
(888) 999-7440; or e-mail: care@life-flo.com

Maker of Progestacare.

Neways
150 E 400 North
PO Box 651
Salem, UT 84653
(801) 423-2800

A multilevel marketing (MLM) company, they make Endau progesterone cream.

Products of Nature
54 Danbury Rd
Ridgefield, CT 06877
(800) 665-5952

Maker of Natural Woman progesterone cream.

Sarati International
Rte 3 Box 385
Ted Hunt Rd
Los Fresno, TX 78566
(956) 233-5001

Maker of Pro-Osteo-All, Estro-All cream, and Natural Progesterone Cream.

Springboard for Health
2801 Salinas Hwy., Bldg. F Monterey, CA 93940
(800) 662-8045

A multi-level marketing company (MLM), ProBalance.

THG Health Products
P.O. Box 97
Oxford, PA 19363, (888) 623-4372, (610) 998-1080
ProCreme.

Transitions for Health, Inc.
621 SW Alder Ste 900
Portland, OR 97205-3627
(503) 226-1010 or (800) 648-8211
Web site (www.progest.com)

Maker of Pro-Gest and Emerita.

SALIVARY HORMONE TESTING

Aeron Life Cycles
1933 Davis St Ste 310
San Leandro, CA 94577
(800) 631-7900

Great Smokies Diagnostic Lab
63 Zillicoa St
Asheville, NC 28801
(800) 522-4762 (for doctors) or (888) 891-3061 (for consumers)

David Zava
ZRT Laboratory
12505 NW Cornell Rd
Portland, OR 97213
(503) 469-0741

HOW TO GET AN AMAS TEST

To get a free AMAS test kit, call Oncolab at (800) 922-8378. Leave your name, address, and phone number. They will send you a kit to bring to your doctor, who will sign the enclosed forms and direct you to a lab that will draw your blood and send it to Oncolab.

HOW TO GET A FERTILITY AWARENESS MINI-MICROSCOPE

Write for more information to CycleView Info, PO Box 84900, Phoenix, AZ 85071, or call (800) 528-0559. It costs $39.95 and comes with an instructional video and cycle chart.

HOW TO FIND A HEALTH CARE PROFESSIONAL IN YOUR AREA WHO USES NATURAL HORMONES

Of course we can't guarantee that any given individual you might contact is knowledgeable, competent, and will work in partnership with you, but these resources will give you a good jump-start on your search. One of the best sources of information is your local health food store.

Organizations you can contact that will give you a referral in your area are:

American College for Advancement in Medicine
PO Box 3427

Laguna Hills, CA 92654

Send a self-addressed envelope with postage for two
ounces, or visit their Web site at www.acam.org

American Association of Naturopathic Physicians
601 Valley St Ste 105
Seattle, WA 98109
(206) 298-0126

Send $5 for a National Referral Directory and brochure,
or fax your request with credit card information to
(206) 298-0129. You can also visit their Web site at
www.naturopathic.org/welcome.html.

American Preventive Medicine Assoc.
PO Box 458
Great Falls, VA 22066
(703) 759-0662

NATURAL PEST CONTROL

The Bio-Integral Resource Center
PO Box 7414
Berkeley, CA 94707
(510) 524-2567

A nonprofit educational organization that provides information and services in the area of "least-toxic" pest control, also known as integrated pest management (IPM).

Rachel Carson Council, Inc.
8940 Jones Mill Rd
Chevy Chase, MD 20815

Provides information on pesticides and chemicals and publishes a newsletter. An excellent source of low-cost books and pamphlets on natural lawns and gardens.

Northwest Coalition for Alternatives to Pesticides (NCAP)
PO Box 1393
Eugene, OR 97440
(503) 344-5044

An information service on the hazards of pesticides and alternatives to their use. Offers information packets, books, and a newsletter and has an extensive library.

National Coalition against the Misuse of Pesticides (NCAMP)
701 E St SE
Washington, DC 20003
(202) 543-5450

A voice for pesticide safety and alternatives. Publishes a quarterly newsletter and has a good list of books and pamphlets.

EXERCISE

Find a reputable trainer in your area by calling the American College of Sports Medicine (ACSM) at (317) 637-

9200 or the National Academy of Sports Medicine (NASM) at (800) 656-2739.

If you're hiring a gym trainer, be sure the gym trainer's certified by one of these organizations or by the American Council of Exercise.

Recommended Reading

―――――――――― ❖ ――――――――――

Cleansing, Fasting, Detoxification

Astor, Stephen. *Hidden Food Allergies.* Garden City, N.Y.: Avery Publishing, 1988.

Bland, Jeffrey, Ph.D. *The 20-Day Rejuvenation Diet Program.* New Canaan, Conn.: Keats Publishing, 1997.

Blaylock, Russell. *Excitotoxins: The Taste That Kills.* Santa Fe, N.M.: Health Press, 1994.

Calbom, Cherie, and Maureen Keane. *Juicing for Life.* Garden City, N.Y.: Avery Publishing, 1992.

Golan, Ralph, M.D. *Optimal Wellness.* New York: Ballantine Books, 1995.

Walker, Morton. *The Chelation Way.* Garden City, N.Y.: Avery Publishing, 1990.

Creating a Toxin-Free Environment

Schultz, Warren. *The Chemical-Free Lawn: The Newest Varieties and Techniques to Grow Lush, Hardy Grass with No Pesticides, No Herbicides, No Chemical Fertilizers*. Emmaus, Pa.: Rodale Press.

Steinman, David, and Michael R. Wisner. *Living Healthy in a Toxic World*. New York: Perigee Books, 1996.

Steinman, David. *Diet for a Poisoned Planet: How to Choose Safe Foods for You and Your Family*. New York: Ballantine Books, 1990.

Women's Health

Boston Women's Health Book Collective. *The New Our Bodies, Ourselves*. New York: Simon & Schuster, 1992.

Coney, Sandra. *The Menopause Industry*. Alameda, Calif.: Hunter House, 1994.

DeMarco, Carolyn, M.D. *Take Charge of Your Body*. Aurora, Ontario: Well-Woman Press, 1996.

Love, Susan. *Dr. Susan Love's Breast Book*. Redding, Mass.: Addison-Wesley, 1990.

Northrup, Christiane, M.D. *Women's Bodies, Women's Wisdom*. New York: Bantam Books, 1994.

Owens, Lara. *Honoring Menstruation—A Time of Self-Renewal*. Freedom, CA: Crossing Press, 1998.

Peat, Raymond. *From PMS to Menopause: Female Hormones in Context*, Eugene, Ore.: Raymond Peat, 1997.

Alternative Medicine and Nutrition

Batmanghelidj, F., M.D. *Your Body's Many Cries for Water*. Falls Church, Va.: Global Health Solutions, 1995.

D'Adamo, Peter, N.D. *Eat Right 4 Your Type.* New York: Putnam, 1996.

Fallon, Sally, *Nourishing Traditions.* San Diego, Calif.: ProMotion Publishing, 1995.

Galland, Leo, M.D. *The Four Pillars of Healing.* New York: Random House, 1997.

Golan, Ralph, M.D. *Optimal Wellness.* New York: Ballantine Books, 1995.

Jahnke, Roger. *The Healer Within.* San Francisco: Harper Collins, 1997.

Lown, Bernard. *The Lost Art of Healing.* Boston: Houghton Mifflin, 1996.

Mindell, Earl, R.Ph., Ph.D., and Virginia Hopkins. *Dr. Earl Mindell's What You Should Know About* series. New Canaan, Conn.: Keats Publishing, 1996.

————. *Prescription Alternatives.* New Canaan, Conn.: Keats Publishing, 1998.

Morton, Mary, and Michael Morton. *Five Steps to Selecting the Best Alternative Medicine.* Novato, Calif.: New World Library, 1996.

Myss, Caroline. *Anatomy of the Spirit.* New York: Random House, 1997.

Pizzorno, Joseph N. *Total Wellness.* Rocklin, Calif.: Prima Publishing, 1996.

Robbins, John. *Reclaiming Our Health.* Tiburon, Calif.: H.J. Kramer, 1996.

Rose, Marc, M.D. and Michael Rose, M.D. *Save Your Sight.* New York: Warner Books, 1998.

Sears, Barry. *The Zone.* New York: HarperCollins, 1996.

Todd, Gary Price, M.D. *Nutrition, Health and Disease.* West Chester, Pa.: Whitford Press, 1985.

Hormones

Barnes, Broda. *Hypothyroidism: The Unsuspected Illness.* New York: Harper & Row, 1976.

Khalsa, Dharma Singh, M.D. *Brain Longevity.* New York: Warner Books, 1997.

Lee, John R., M.D., with Virginia Hopkins. *What Your Doctor May Not Tell You about Menopause: The Breakthrough Book on Natural Progesterone.* New York: Warner Books, 1996.

Sahelian, Ray. *DHEA: A Practical Guide*, Avery Publishing, Garden City, N.Y.: 1996.

———. *Pregnenolone: A Practical Guide.* Marina del Rey, Calif.: Melatonin/DHEA Research Institute, 1996.

Drugs

Breggin, Peter. *Talking Back to Prozac.* New York: St. Martin's Press, 1994.

Fried, Stephen. *Bitter Pills: Inside the Hazardous World of Legal Drugs.* New York: Bantam Books, 1998.

Lappe, Marc. *When Antibiotics Fail: Restoring the Ecology of the Body.* Berkeley, Calif.: North Atlantic Books, 1995.

Schmidt, Michael, Lendon Smith, and Keith Sehnert. *Beyond Antibiotics.* Berkeley, Calif.: North Atlantic Books, 1994.

Children

Lappe, Marc. *When Antibiotics Fail: Restoring the Ecology of the Body.* Berkeley, Calif.: North Atlantic Books, 1995.

Schmidt, Michael, Lendon Smith, and Keith Sehnert. *Beyond Antibiotics.* Berkeley, Calif.: North Atlantic Books, 1994.

Smith, Lendon, M.D. *How to Raise a Healthy Child.* New York: M. Evans & Co., 1996.

Zand, Janet, O.M.D., Rachel Walton, R.N., and Robert Rountree, M.D. *A Parent's Guide to Medical Emergencies.* Garden City, N.Y.: Avery Publishing, 1997.

Exercise

Andes, Karen. *A Woman's Book of Strength.* Perigee Books, 1995.

Protugues, Gladys, and Joyce Vedral. *Hard Bodies.* Dell Paperbacks, 1997.

References

❖

(Because so many of the references listed are relevant throughout the book, this is an alphabetized listing of all references used. Whenever practical, we have used the name of the author of the study in the book, to make it easy to look up here.)

Adams, M. R. et al. "Medroxyprogesterone Acetates Antagonize Inhibitory Effects of Conjugated Equine Estrogens on Common Artery Atherosclerosis." *Arterioscler Thromb Vasc Biol* 17(1) (January 1997): 217–21.

"Advance Report of Final Natality Statistics." *Monthly Vital Statistics Report* 42(3) (1993).

Andrews, R. V. "Influence of Adrenal Gland on Gonadal Function." In *Advances in Sex Hormone Research,* edited by R. A. Thomas and R. L. Singhal. *Volume 3* of *Regulatory Mechanisms Affecting Gonadal Hormone Action.* (Baltimore: University Park, 1976): 197–215.

Arafat, E. S., and J. T. Hargrove. "Sedative and Hypnotic Effects of Oral Administration of Micronized Progesterone May Be Mediated through Its Metabolites." *American Journal of Obstetrics and Gynecology* 159 (1988): 1203–1209.

Asch, R. H., and R. Greenblatt. "Steroidogenesis in the Postmenopausal Ovary." *Clinical Obstetrics and Gynecology* 4(1) (1977): 85.

Ashcroft, G. S. et al. "Estrogen Accelerates Cutaneous Wound Healing Associated with an Increase in TGF-beta 1 Levels." *Nature Medicine* 3 (1997): 11.

Astrow, A. B. "St. Vincent's Hospital and Medical Center." *Lancet* 343 (1994): 495.

Aufrere, M.B. et al. "Progesterone: an Overview and Recent Advances." *J Pharmaceut Sci* 65 (1976): 783.

Backstrom, T. "Epileptic Seizure in Women Related to Plasma Oestrogen and Progesterone during the Menstrual Cycle." *Acta Neurol Scand* 54 (1976): 321–347.

Backstrom, T. et al. "Estrogen and Progesterone in Plasma in Relation to Premenstrual Tension." *J Steroid Biochem Mol Biol* 5 (1974): 257–260.

————. "Effects of Ovarian Steroid Hormones on Brain Excitability and Their Relation to Epilepsy Seizure Variation during the Menstrual Cycle." *Advances in Epileptology. Fifteenth Epilepsy International Symposium.* New York: Raven Press.

Bayer, S. R. et al. "Clinical Manifestations and Treatment of Dysfunctional Uterine Bleeding." *Journal of the American Medical Association* 269 (1993): 1823–1828.

Beumont P.J.L. et al. "Luteinizing Hormone and Progesterone Levels after Hysterectomy." *British Medical Journal* 836 (1972): 363.

Beynon, H.I.C., N. D. Garbett, and P. J. Barnes. "Severe Premenstrual Exacerbations of Asthma; Effect of Intramuscular Progesterone." *Lancet* (1988): 370–371.

Bloom, T., A. Ojanotko-Harri, M. Laine, and I. Huhtaniemi. "Metabolism of Progesterone and Testosterone in Human Parotid and Submandibular Salivary Glands in Vitro." *J Steroid Biochem Mol Biol* 44(1) (January 1993): 69–76.

Bourgain, C. et al. "Effects of Natural Progesterone on the Morphology of the Endometrium in Patients with Primary Ovarian Failure." *Human Reproduction* 5 (1990): 537–543.

Bower, B. "Stress Hormones May Speed Up Brain Aging." *Science News* 153(17) (1998): 263.

Bowman, K. et al. "The Influence of Progesterone and Androgens on the Growth of Endometrial Carcinoma." *Cancer* 71(11) (June 1, 1993): 3565–3569.

Burke, G. L. "The Potential Use of a Dietary Soy Supplement as a Postmenopausal Hormone Replacement Therapy." Abstract from the Second International Symposium on the Role of Soy in Preventing and Treating Chronic Disease, Brussels, Belgium, 1996.

Businco L. et al. "Allergenicity and Nutritional Adequacy of Soy Protein Formulas." *Journal of Pediatrics* 121 (1992): S21–S28.

Campbell, B. C., and P. T. Ellison. "Menstrual Variation in Salivary Testosterone among Regularly Cycling

Women." *Hormone Research* (Switzerland) 37(4–5) (1992): 132–136.

Campbell, W. W. et al. "Increased Energy Requirements and Changes in Body Composition with Resistance Training in Older Adults." *American Journal of Clinical Nutrition* 60(2) (1994): 167–175.

Cavalieri, E. L., D. E. Stack, P. D. Devanesan, R. Todorovic et al. "Molecular Origin of Cancer: Catechol Estrogen-3,4-quinones as Endogenous Tumor Initiators." *Proc Natl Acad Sci* 94 (1997): 10937–10942.

Centerwall, B. S. "Premenopausal Hysterectomy and Cardiovascular Disease." *American Journal of Obstetrics and Gynecology* 139 (1981): 58–61.

Chang, K. J., T.T.Y. Lee, G. Linares-Cruz, S. Fournier, and B. de Lingieres. "Influences of Percutaneous Administration of Estradiol and Progesterone on Human Breast Epithelial Cell Cycle in Vivo." *Fertility and Sterility* 63 (1995): 785–791.

Christ, J. E. et al. "The Residual Ovary Syndrome." *Obstetrics & Gynecology* 46 (1975): 551–556.

Clark, G. M., and W. L. McQuire. "Progesterone Receptors and Human Breast Cells." *Breast Cancer Research and Treatment* 3 (1983): 157–163.

Collins, P. et al. "Estrogen Replacement Therapy and Exercise Performance in Postmenopausal Women with Coronary Artery Disease." *American Journal of Cardiology* 81(2) (January 15, 1998): 259–260.

Corvol, P. et al. "Effect of Progesterone and Progestins on Water and Salt Metabolism." *Progesterone and Progestins.* New York: Raven Press, 1983.

Cowan, L. D., L. Gordis, J. A. Tonascia, and G. S. Jones. "Breast Cancer Incidence in Women with a History of Progesterone Deficiency." *American Journal of Epidemiology* 114 (1981): 209–217.

Cramer, S. R., D. C. Nieman, and J. W. Lee. "The Effects of Moderate Exercise Training on Psychological Well-Being and Mood State in Women." *Psychosomatic Research* 35 (1991): 437–439.

Cranton, E., and W. Fryer. *Resetting the Clock.* New York: M. Evans and Co., 1996.

Cummings, S. R. et al. "Risk Factors for Hip Fracture in White Women." *New England Journal of Medicine* 332 (1995): 767–773.

Dalton, K. "The Aetiology of Premenstrual Syndrome Is with the Progesterone Receptors." *Medical Hypotheses* 31 (1987): 321–327.

———. "Erythema Multiforme Associated with Menstruation." *Journal of the Royal Society of Medicine* 78 (1985): 787–788.

———. "Influence of Menstruation on Glaucoma." *British Journal of Ophthalmology* 51(10) (1967): 692–695.

———. *Premenstrual Syndrome.* London: Heinemann, 1964.

———. *The Premenstrual Syndrome and Progesterone Therapy.* 2nd ed. London: Heinemann, 1984.

———. "Progesterone Suppositories and Pessaries in the Treatment of Menstrual Migraine." *Headache* 12 (1973): 151–159.

Darcy, K. M., S. F. Shoemaker, P. H. Lee, B. A. Ganis,

and M. Margot. "Hydrocortisone and Progesterone Regulation of the Proliferation, Morphogenesis, and Functional Differentiation of Normal Rat Mammary Epithelial Cells in Three-Dimensional Primary Culture." *Journal of Cellular Physiology* 163 (1995): 365–379.

Davis, D. L., H. L. Bradlow, M. Wolff, T. Woodruff, D. G. Hoel, and H. Anton-Culver. "Medical Hypothesis: Xenohormones as Preventable Causes of Breast Cancer." *Environmental Health Perspectives* 101 (1993): 372–377.

DeBold, J. F., and C. A. Frye. "Progesterone and the Neural Mechanisms of Hamster Sexual Behavior." *Psychoneuroendocrinology* 19 (1994): 563–579.

Dennerstein, L., C. Spencer-Gardner, J. B. Brown, M. A. Smith, and G. D. Burrows. "Premenstrual Tension—Hormone Profiles." *J Psychosomat Obstet Gynaec* 3 (1984): 37–51.

Dennerstein, L. et al. "Progesterone and the Premenstrual Syndrome: A Double-Blind Crossover Trial." *British Medical Journal* 290 (1985): 1017–1021.

Devroey, P., G. Palermo et al. "Progesterone Administration in Patients with Absent Ovaries." *International Journal of Fertility* 34 (1990): 188–193.

Eliasson, O., and H. H. Scherzer. "Recurrent Respiratory Failure in Premenstrual Asthma." *Connecticut Med* 12 (1984): 777–778.

Ellison, P. T. "Measurements of Salivary Progesterone." *Annals of the New York Academy of Sciences* 694 (September 20, 1993): 161–176.

Ellison, P. T., S. F. Lipson, M. T. O'Rourke, G. R. Bentley, A. M. Harrigan, C. Painter-Brick, and V. J. Vizthum. "Population Variation in Ovarian Function" (letter). *Lancet* 342(8868) (August 14, 1993): 433–434.

Ellison, P. T., C. Painter-Brick, S. F. Lipson, and M. T. O'Rourke. "The Ecological Context of Human Ovarian Function." *Human Reproduction* 8(12) (December 1993): 2248–2258.

Fallon, S. W., and M. G. Enig. "Soy Products for Dairy Products? Not So Fast." *Health Freedom News,* September 1995.

Ferguson, E. L. et al. "Dietary Calcium, Phytate, and Zinc Intakes and the Calcium, Phytate, and Zinc Molar Ratios of the Diets of a Selected Group of East African Children." *American Journal of Clinical Nutrition* 50(6) (1989): 1450–1456.

Formby, B., and T. S. Wiley. "Progesterone Inhibits Growth and Induces Apoptosis in Breast Cancer Cells: Inverse Effect on Expression of p53 and Bcl-2." Sansum Medical Research Foundation, Santa Barbara, Calif., 1997.

Gambrell, R. D. "Use of Progestogens in Post-Menopausal Women." *International Journal of Fertility* 34 (1989): 315–321.

Garcia, C. R., and W. Cutler. "Preservation of the Ovary: A Reevaluation," *Fertility and Sterility* 42(4) (1985): 510–514.

Gibbs, C. J., I. I. Coutts, R. Lock, O. S. Finnegan, and

R. J. White. "Premenstrual Exacerbation of Asthma."
Thorax 39 (1984): 833–836.

Gillet, J. Y. "Induction of Amenorrhea during Hormone
Replacement Therapy: Optimal Micronized Progesterone Doses: A Multicenter Study." *Maturitas* 19
(1994): 103–116.

Gompel, A., C. Malet, P. Spritzer, J.-P. La Lardrie et al.
"Progestin Effect on Cell Proliferation and 17ß-
hydroxysteroid Dehydrogenase Activity in Normal
Human Breast Cells in Culture." *Journal of Clinical
Endocrinology and Metabolism* 63 (1986): 1174.

Gompel, A., J. C. Sabourin, A. Martin, H. Yaneva et al.
"Bcl-2 Expression in Normal Endometrium during
the Menstrual Cycle." *American Journal of Pathology*
144 (1994): 1196–1202.

Gray, L. A. "The Use of Progesterone in Nervous Tension States." *Southern Medical Journal* 34 (1941):
1004.

Greene, R., and K. Dalton. "The Premenstrual Syndrome." *British Medical Journal* 1 (1953):
1007–1011.

Hammond, C. B., and W. S. Maxson. *Physiology of the
Menopause.* New York: Upjohn Co., 1983.

Hanley, S. P., "Asthma Variations with Menstruation."
British J Dis Chest 75 (1981): 306–308.

Harris, B., L. Lovett, R. G. Newcombe, G. F. Read, R.
Walker, and D. Riad-Fahmy. "Maternity Blues and
Major Endocrine Changes: Cardiff Puerperal Mood
and Hormone Study II (Wales)." *British Medical Journal* April 9, 1994.

Harris, S. et al. "Influence of Body Weight on Rates of Change in Bone Density of the Spine, Hip, and Radius in PostMenopausal Women." *Calcif Tissue Int* 50 (1992): 19–23.

Hata, K. et al, "Effect of Regular Aerobic Exercise on Cerebrovascular Tone in Young Women." *Journal of Ultrasound Medicine* 17(2) (February 1998): 133–136.

Herman-Giddens, M. E., E. J. Slora, R. C. Wasserman, C. J. Bourdony et al. "Secondary Sexual Characteristics and Menses in Young Girls Seen in Office Practice: A Study from the Pediatric Research in Office Settings Network." *Pediatrics* 99 (1997): 505–512.

Herzog, A. G. "Intermittent Progesterone Therapy and Frequency of Complex Partial Seizures in Women with Menstrual Disorders." *Neurology* 36 (1986): 1607–1610.

Hreshchyshn, M. M. et al. "Effects of Natural Menopause, Hysterectomy, and Oophorectomy on Lumbar Spine and Femoral Neck Bone Densities." *Obstetrics & Gynecology* 72 (1988): 631–638.

Hrushesky, W.J.M. "Breast Cancer, Timing of Surgery, and the Menstrual Cycle: Call for Prospective Trial." *Journal of Women's Health* 5 (1996): 555–556.

Inoh, A., K. Kamiya, Y. Fujii, and K. Yokoro. "Protective Effects of Progesterone and Tamoxifen in Estrogen-Induced Mammary Carcinogenesis in Ovariectomized W/Fu Rats." *Japanese Journal of Cancer Research* 76 (1985): 699–704.

Jacobson, J. L., and S. W. Jacobson. "Intellectual Impairment in Children Exposed to Polychlorinated Biphenyls in Utero." *New England Journal of Medicine* 335 (1996): 783–789.

Kandouz, M., M. Siromachkova, D. Jacob, B. C. Marquet et al. "Antagonism between Estradiol and Progestin on Bcl-2 Expression in Breast Cancer Cells." *International Journal of Cancer* 68 (1996): 120–125.

Kushi, L. H. "Physical Activity and Mortality in Postmenopausal Women." *Journal of the American Medical Association* 277(16) (April 1997): 1287–1292.

LaPierre, A. et al. "Exercise and Psychoneuroimmunology." *Medicine and Science in Sports and Exercise* 26(2) (1994): 182–190.

Leis, H. P. "Endocrine Prophylaxis of Breast Cancer with Cyclic Estrogen and Progesterone." *Intern Surg* 45 (1966): 496–503.

Liener, I. E. "Implications of Antinutritional Components in Soybean Foods." *Crit Rev Food Sci Nutr* 34 (1994): 31–67.

Lipsett, M. P. "Steroid Hormones." In *Reproductive Endocrinology, Physiology, and Clinical Management,* edited by S.S.C. Yen and R. B. Jaffe. Philadelphia: W. B. Saunders, 1978.

Lipson, S. F., and P. T. Ellison. "Reference Values for Luteal 'Progesterone' Measured by Salivary Radioimmunoassay." *Fertility and Sterility* 61(3) (March 1994): 448–454.

Lydon, J. P., F. J. DeMayo, O. M. Conneely, and B. W. O'Malley. "Reproductive Phenotypes of the Progesterone Receptor Null Mutant Mouse." *J Steroid Biochem Molec Biol* 56 (1996): 67–77.

Magill, P. J. "Investigation of the Efficacy of Progesterone Pessaries in the Relief of Symptoms of Premenstrual Syndrome." *British Journal of General Practice* (November 1995): 598–593.

Mahesh, V. B., D. W. Brann, and L. G. Hendry. "Diverse Modes of Action of Progesterone and Its Metabolites." *J Steroid Biochem Molec Biol* 56 (1996): 209–219.

Majewska, M. D. "Steroid Hormone Metabolites Are Barbiturate-like Modulators of GABA System." *Science* 232 (1986): 1004–1007.

Matthews, K. A. et al. "Prior to Use of Estrogen Replacement Therapy, Are Users Healthier Than Nonusers?" *American Journal of Epidemiology* 143(10) (1996): 971–978.

McCardle, W. D., F. I. Katch, and V. L. Katch. *Exercise Physiology: Energy, Nutrition, and Human Performance.* Philadelphia: Lea & Febiger, 1991.

McKinlay, S. M. et al, "The Normal Menopause Transition." *Maturitas* 14 (1992): 103–114.

Miyagawa, K., J. Rosch, F. Stanczyk, and K. Hermsmeyer. "Medroxyprogesterone Interferes with Ovarian Steroid Protection Against Coronary Vasospasm." *Nature Medicine* 3 (March 3, 1997): 324–327.

Miles, R. A. "Pharmokinetics and Endometrial Tissue Levels of Progesterone after Administration by Intramuscular and Vaginal Routes: A Comparative Study." *Fertility and Sterility* 62 (1994): 485–490.

Mohr, P. E., D. Y. Wang, W. M. Gregory, M. A. Richards, and I. S. Fentiman. "Serum Progesterone and Prognosis in Operable Breast Cancer." *British Journal of Cancer* 73 (1996): 1552–1555.

Moyer, D. L. et al. "Prevention of Endometrial Hyperplasia by Progesterone during Long-Term Estradiol Replacement: Influence of Bleeding Pattern and Secretory Changes." *Fertility and Sterility* 59 (1993): 992–997.

Munday, M. R. et al. "Correlations between Progesterone, Oestradiol and Aldosterone Levels in the Premenstrual Syndrome." *Clinical Endocrinology* 14 (1981): 1–9.

Nash, M. S. "Exercise and Immunology." *Medicine and Science in Sports and Exercise* 26(2) (February 1994): 125–127.

Nillius, S. J. et al. "Plasma Levels of Progesterone after Vaginal, Rectal or Intramuscular Administration of Progesterone." *American Journal of Obstetrics and Gynecology* 110 (1971): 470–477.

Novak, E. R. et al. "Enzyme Histochemistry of the Menopausal Ovary Associated with Normal and Abnormal Endometrium." *American Journal of Obstetrics and Gynecology* 93 (1965): 669.

O'Brien, P.M.S., C. Selby, and E. M. Symonds. "Progesterone, Fluid and Electrolytes in Premenstrual Syndrome." *British Medical Journal* 1 (1980): 1161–1163.

O'Rourke, M. T., and P. T. Ellison. "Age and Prognosis in Premonopausal Breast Cancer" (letter; comment). *Lancet* 342(8662) (July 3, 1993): 60.

Painter-Brick, C., D. S. Lotstein, and P. T. Ellison. "Seasonality of Reproductive Function and Weight Loss in Rural Nepali Women." *Human Reproduction* 8(5) (May 1993): 684–690.

Pate, R. R. et al. "Physical Activity and Public Health: A Recommendation from the Centers for Disease Control and Prevention and the American College of Sports Medicine." *Journal of the American Medical Association* 273(5) (1995): 402–407.

Petrakis, N. L. et al. "Stimulatory Influence of Soy Protein Isolate on Breast Secretion in Pre- and Postmenopausal Women." *Cancer Epidemiol Biomarkers Prev* 5 (1996): 785–794.

Pujol, P., S. G. Hilsenbeck, G. C. Chamness, and R. M. Elledge. "Rising Levels of Estrogen Receptor in Breast Cancer over 2 Decades." *Cancer* 74 (1994): 1601–1606.

Rannevik G. et al. "A Longitudinal Study of the Perimenopausal Transition: Altered Profiles of Steroid and Pituitary Hormones, SHBG and Bone Mineral Density." *Maturitas* 21 (1995): 103–113.

Ranney, B. et al. "The Future Function and Fortune of Ovarian Tissue which is Retained in Vivo During Hysterectomy." *American Journal of Obstetrics and Gynecology* 128 (1977): 626–634.

Reid, I. R. "Determinants of Total Body and Regional Bone Mineral Density in Normal Postmenopausal Women—A Key Role for Fat Mass." *J Clin Endocrinol Metab* 75 (1992): 45–51.

Reidel, H. H. et al. "Ovarian Failure Phenomena after

Hysterectomy." *Journal of Reproductive Medicine* 31 (1986): 597–600.

Rodriguez Macias, K. A. "Catamenial Epilepsy: Gynecological and Hormonal Implications: Five Case Reports." *Gynecology and Endrocrinology* 10 (1996): 139–142.

Rodriquez, C., E. E. Calle, R. J. Coates, H. L. Miracle-McMahill, M. J. Thun, and C. W. Heath. "Estrogen Replacement Therapy and Fatal Ovarian Cancer." *American Journal of Epidemiology* 141 (1995): 828–834.

Rubinow, D. R., M. C. Hoban, G. N. Grover, D. S. Galloway, P. Roy-Byrne, R. Andersen, and G. R. Merriam. "Changes in Plasma Hormones across the Menstrual Cycle in Patients with Menstrually Related Mood Disorders and in Control Subjects." *American Journal of Obstetrics and Gynecology* 158 (1988): 5–11.

Rylance, P. B. et al. "Natural Progesterone and Antihypertensive Action." *British Medical Journal* 290 (1985): 13–14.

Sabourin, J. C., A. Martin, J. Baruch, J. B. True et al. "Bcl-2 Expression in Normal Breast Tissue during the Menstrual Cycle." *International Journal of Cancer* 59 (1994): 1–6.

Sampson, G. A. "Premenstrual Syndrome: A Double-Blind Controlled Trial of Progesterone and Placebo." *British Journal of Psychiatry* 135 (1979): 209.

Sandstrom, B. et al. "Absorption of Zinc from Soy Protein Meals in Humans." *Journal of Nutrition* 117 (1987): 321–327.

Santell, R. C. et al. "Dietary Genistein Exerts Estrogenic

Effects upon the Uterus, Mammary Gland and the Hypothalamic/Pituitary Axis in Rats." *Journal of Nutrition* 127(2) (February 1997): 263–269.

Schmidt, Peter J. et al. "Differential Behavioral Effects of Gonadal Steroids in Women with and in Those without Premenstrual Syndrome." *New England Journal of Medicine* 338 (1998): 209–216.

Seppa, N. "Even Fraternal Twins May Share Cancer Risk." *Science News* 152 (December 1997): 389.

Shi-Zhong, B., Y. De-Ling, R. Xiu-Hai, J. Li-Zhen et al. "Progesterone Induces Apoptosis and Up-Regulation of p53 Expression in Human Ovarian Carcinoma Cell Lines." *American Cancer Society* (1997): 1944–1950.

Siddle, N. et al. "The Effect of Hysterectomy on the Age at Ovarian Failure: Identification of a Subgroup of Women with Premature Loss of Ovarian Function and Literature Review." *Fertility and Sterility* 47 (1987): 94–100.

Simon, J. A. "Micronized Progesterone: Vaginal and Oral Uses." *Clinical Obstetrics and Gynecology* 38(4) (1995): 902–914.

Sitruk-Ware, R. et al. "Oral Micronized Progesterone." *Contraception* 36 (1987): 373.

Snow-Harter, C. M. "Bone Health and Prevention of Osteoporosis in Active and Athletic Women." *Clinics in Sports Medicine* 13(2) (April 1994): 389–404.

Steinberg, K. K. et al. "Sex Steroids and Bone Density in Premenopausal and Perimenopausal Women." *J Clin Endocrinol Metab* 69 (1989): 553–559.

Stone, S. C. et al. "The Acute Effect of Hysterectomy on

Ovarian Function." *American Journal of Obstetrics and Gynecology* 121 (1975): 193–197.

Sulak, P. J. "The Perimenopause: A Critical Time in a Woman's Life." *International Journal of Fertility* 41(2) (1996): 85–89.

Thompson, H. J. "Effects of Physical Activity and Exercise on Experimentally Induced Mammary Carcinogenesis." *Breast Cancer Research and Treatment* 46 (2–3) (November 1997): 135–141.

Tzourio, C. et al. "Case-Controlled Study of Migraine and Risk of Ischemic Stroke in Young Women." *British Medical Journal* 310 (1995): 830–833.

Ursin, G. "Oral Contraceptive Use and Adenocarcinoma of Cervix." *Lancet* 344(8934) (1994): 1390–1394.

Vitzthum, V. J., M. von Dornum, and P. T. Ellison. "Brief Communication: Effect of Coca-Leaf Chewing on Salivary Progesterone Assays." *American Journal of Physical Anthropology* 92(4) (December 1993): 539–544.

Watson, N. R., and J.W.W. Studd. "Bone Loss Following Hysterectomy with Ovarian Conservation." *European Journal of Obstetrics, Gynecology and Reproductive Biology* 49 (1993): 87.

Weinberg, R. A. "How Cancer Arises." *Scientific American* (September 1996): 62–70.

Wen, X. L. et al. "Effects of Adrenocorticotropic Hormone, Human Chorionic Gonadotropin, and Insulin on Steroid Production by Human Adrenocortical Carcinoma Cells in Culture." *Cancer Research* 45(8) (August 1985): 3974–3978.

White, R. F., and S. P. Proctor. "Solvents and Neurotoxicity." *Lancet* 349 (1997): 1239–1243.

Wilgus, H. S., Jr. et al. "Goitrogenicity of Soybeans." *Journal of Nutrition* 22 (1941): 45–52.

Williams, P. T. "Relationships of Heart Disease Risk Factors to Exercise Quantity and Intensity." *Archives of Internal Medicine* 158(3) (1998): 237–245.

Witt, D. M., J. Young, and D. Crews. "Progesterone and Sexual Behavior in Males." *Psychoneuroendocrinology* 19 (1994): 553–562.

Wojnarowska, F. et al. "Progesterone-Induced Erythema Multiform." *Journal of the Royal Society of Medicine* 78 (1987): 407–81.

Wolk, A. et al. "A Prospective Study of Association of Monounsaturated Fat and Other Types of Fat with Risk of Breast Cancer." *Archives of Internal Medicine* 158 (1998): 41–45.

Writing Group for the PEPI Trial. "Effects of Estrogen or Estrogen/Progestin Regimens on Heart Disease Risk Factors in Postmenopausal Women: The Postmenopausal Estrogen/Progestin Interventions." *Journal of the American Medical Association* 273 (1995): 199–208.

Zava, D. T., and G. Duwe. "Estrogenic and Antiproliferative Properties of Genistein and Other Flavonoids in Human Breast Cancer Cells in Vitro." *Nutrition and Cancer* 27 (1997): 31–40.

Bibliography

Colborn, Theo, et al. *Our Stolen Future*. New York: Penguin Books, 1997.

Grant, Ellen. *The Bitter Pill: How Safe Is the Perfect Contraceptive?* London: Elm Tree Books, 1985.

Jefferies, W. McK. *Safe Uses of Cortisone*. Springfield, Ill.: Charles C. Thomas, 1981.

Jones, Howard W. III, Anne Colston Wentz, and Lonnie S. Burnett, eds. *Novak's Textbook of Gynecology*. 11th ed. Baltimore: Williams & Wilkins, 1988.

Sheehy, Gail. *The Silent Passage*. Rev. ed. New York: Pocket Books, 1998.

Tietz, Norbert W., Ph.D., ed. *Textbook of Clinical Chemistry*. Philadelphia: W. B. Saunders Co., 1986.

Thomas, J. Hywel, and Brian Gilham, eds. *Will's Biochemical Basis of Medicine*. 2d ed. London: Wright of London, 1989.

Index

Pages of illustrations appear in italics.

Adams, M. R., 81
Adenosine triphosphate (ATP), 208
Adrenal glands: exhausted, 16–17,
    54, 163–72; healing, 171–72,
    278; progesterone cream for,
    170, 171; rest for, 171; stressed,
    55, 150; symptoms of
    insufficiency, 167–68, 278; what
    to avoid, 172. *See also* Cortisol
Aging: estrogen dominance and, 51;
    estrogen therapy and, 57
Alcohol, 16
Allergy, 51, 156, 222, 310–14
Alzheimer's disease, 58, 109
AMAS test, 125–26, 230
Androgen dominance, 126, 135
Androstenedione, 25, 27, 211,
    383–84
Anovulation, 54
Anxiety, 29, 54, 79, 156, 222
Arthritis, 53
Asthma, 53, 167, 311

Astrow, A. B., 231
Autoimmune disorders, 198–99;
    estrogen dominance and, 51, 68;
    xenohormones and, 98–99

Balance, restoring and maintaining,
    270–83; case history, early
    menopause, 281–83; case history,
    ovarian cysts and need for
    balanced life, 13–17; case history,
    woman athlete, 269–73; clues to
    personal state of well–being,
    277–79; self-care, 273–77;
    symptoms and listening to your
    body, 279–83
Beta carotene, 223, 324–25, 335
Billings, Evelyn and John, 224
Bioflavonoids, 115
Birkmayer, Georg, 209
Birth control implant, 76–78,
    219–20
Birth control options, safe, 224–25

Birth control pill: birth defects and birth marks in children of users, 221; endometriosis treatment, 23–25; health risks, 23, 129, 155, 219–25; irregular bleeding and, 185; nutrient levels, 224; PMS and, 146; premenopausal treatment, 63–64; progestin, 23, 59, 78; urinary tract problems and, 58, 59, 222

Birth control shot (Depo-Provera), 219, 222

Bitter Pill, The: How Safe Is the Perfect Contraceptive (Grant), 189

Bloating. See Water retention

Blood: clots, 51, 67, 110; pressure, high, 63, 110, 166, 167, 169, 221; pressure, low, 169; sugar levels, 55, 67, 165

Bogoch, Samuel and Eleanor, 230

Boman, K., 260

Bones: cortisol and, 34; estrogen dominance and, 51, 68; estrogen therapy for, 59; fluoride and, 35; progesterone and, 34, 68

Borage oil, 153, 154, 187, 334

Boron, 330

Brain: estrogen dominance and, 58, 215; pituitary tumors, 152, 222; progesterone effects, 75–76

Breast cancer: age of onset, 239–40; basics about, 231; birth control pills and, 222; bra types and, 255; case history, alternative treatment, 226–28; case history, progesterone cream, 251; emotional side of, 253–55; facts and figures, 237–40; estriol protection, 59; estrogen

dominance and 51, 68, 180; estrogen receptors and, 33; mammography, 229; massage, 255–56; pregnancy and, 246; prevention program, Dr. Lee's, 256–58; progesterone protective of, 67, 234–37, 238, 239; 243, 244–45, 250, 251; self-exam for, 228; sex hormones and, 240–47, 242; surgery and progesterone levels, 235, 258; treatment, 229–30, 250–53; unopposed estrogen and, 128, 179; xenohormones and, 95, 98, 189–90, 237–38

Breast, fibrocystic or sore and lumpy, 3, 4, 9, 254, ; adrenal exhaustion and, 167; estrogen dominance and, 51, 55, 56, 67, 94; healing, 179–82; massage for, 255; PMS and, 144–46; progesterone cream to treat, 61–62, 179, 367–68; progesterone effects, 67; progestin and, 78–79; unopposed estrogen (HRT) and, 110; what to avoid, 181–82; xenohormones and, 98

Breast swelling or enlargement, 56, 74–75

Caffeine, 172, 1812, 188, 201. See also Coffee

Calcium, 330–31

Cancer: basics about, 228–29; birth control pills and, 221; cell death, programmed, 232; cell differentiation and proliferation, 232–33; diet and, 248–50;

estrogen and, 49, 60, 68, 104, 233, 237–40, 248–49, *249*; genes and, 246–47; hormone-related, 56, 60, 190; phytochemicals found in foods and anticancer actions, 308; test, 125, 229–31; unopposed estrogen (HRT) and, 110; vaginal, 189–90; xenoestrogens and, 53, 94, 97, 250. *See also* Breast cancer; Cervical dysplasia; Endometrial cancer; Prostate cancer; Uterus, cancer

Castor oil pack, 112

Cavalieri, Ercole, 48, 248–49, *249*, 250

Cell, oxygen levels, 68

Cervical dysplasia, 5, 222; cancer and, 221; estrogen dominance and, 51; HRT and, 11; progesterone cream to treat, 62; unopposed estrogen and, 179

Chang, K. J., 241–42, 356

Chinese medicine, 15–17, 20

Cholesterol, 26, 28, 167

Chromium, 331

Chronic fatigue syndrome, 55, 208–9

Clomid, 192

Coffee, 15, 112, 194. *See also* Caffeine

Colburn, Theo, 94

Colds and flu prevention, 335

Collins, Peter, 81

Constipation, 79. 309

Copper, 331–32; estrogen dominance and, 51, 67–68, 331; excess, 156–57, 213–17; progesterone effects, 67

Cortisols, 26, 27, 64, 163; bone growth inhibition, 34; fatigue and, 165–68, 172; health risks, 28–29, 379; PMS and, 145, 150–51; stress and, 28, 155, 359–60; supplementing, 378–81; symptoms of too much, 165; water retention, 36

Cowan, L. D., 234

Dalton, Katherina, 146, 191

Davis, Devra Lee, 95–96

DeMarco, Carolyn, 115–16

Depression: adrenal insufficiency, 167–68; birth control pills and, 224; copper and, 156; estrogen and, 28, 48, 51, 56, 67–68; ovary removal and, 128; premenopause and, 4, 9, 11; progesterone effects, 67; progestin and, 78; synthetic hormones and, 11; zinc-copper connection, 214–17

DES, 93, 189

DHEA, 25–26, 27, 199, 208; supplement, 20, 167, 171, 211, 372, 375–77; wild yam scam and, 44

Diabetes, 32

Diarrhea, 79, 156

Diet and nutrition, 284–336; anti-cancer, 248–50, 255; anti-candidiasis, 320; building blocks of good nutrition, 288–92; carbohydrate and sugar habit, 294–99; carbohydrates, complex, 287–88; case history, college and junk food, 296; case history, food allergy, 310–14; elimination (to

Diet and nutrition (*cont.*)
   detect food allergy), 195,
      314–17; exclusion of dairy,
      106–7, 112, 143, 172, 181, 186,
      304; exclusion of feedlot meat,
      87, 112, 143, 162, 172, 181,
      186, 189, 304–5; fats and oils,
      153–55, 299–303; fiber, 309–10;
      Hanley, Virginia, personal
      history, 291–92; high
      carbohydrate, low–fat, 287; high
      fiber and vegetable-based, 20,
      107, 161, 188, 288, 306–8;
      high-protein, high-fat, 288;
      irregular periods and, 185;
      organic foods, 304–6; ovarian
      cyst and, 126–27;
      phytochemicals found in foods
      and anticancer actions, 308;
      PMS and, 150, 155–57;
      processed foods, 292; soy
      products, 39, 45, 306–7;
      trans–fatty acids (hydrogenated
      oils), avoiding, 152–55, 250,
      301–3; water intake, 20
Dieting, and anovulation, 54
Digestive problems and heartburn,
      9, 15, 222, 317–19, 322
Diosgenin. *See* Wild yam
Douching for yeast infections, 197,
      198
Drug companies: estrogen research
      and, 56–60; synthetic hormones,
      reason for, 25

Eating disorders, 156–57
Echinacea, 335
Elderberry, 335
Ellison, Peter, 237

Emotions: anger, 24, 145, 157–58,
      159, 215; disconnection from, 4;
      hormone balance and, 28, 29;
      PMS and, 157–60
Endometrial cancer, 51, 68, 103,
      104, 221, 252, 259–61
Endometriosis, 4, 55, 104, 211–13;
      birth control pills to treat,
      23–24; case history, 23–25;
      estrogen effects, 67; healing, 214;
      progesterone cream for, 214,
      366–67; progesterone effects, 67,
      213; what to avoid, 214
Environmental toxins and hormone
      imbalance, 26–27, 30, 35, 38,
      84–100, 150, 303–6. *See also*
      Xenohormones
Essential fatty acids (EFAs),
      153–55, 156, 248, 300–303
Estradiol, 27, 49, 245, 250;
      comparison of xenohormones
      with, *91*
Estriol, 27, 49, 59, 210, 257
Estrogen(s), 48–60; benefits
      promised by drug companies, 56,
      109–10; body, effects on, 49;
      brain, effect on, 29; cancer and,
      49, 59, 68, 103–4, 233, 237–40,
      248–49, *249*; cell growth
      stimulation, 49, 50; emotions,
      effect on, 29; lowering levels,
      359–60; manufactured in fat
      cells, 27, 59, 233; manufactured,
      post–menopausal, 139–40;
      receptors, 32, 68, 233; research,
      56–60; unopposed, banning,
      258–59
Estrogen deficiency, 16; depression

and, 29; symptoms, 48, 58; treatment, 58

Estrogen dominance (excess): causes, 52–56, 53, 84–100; deficiencies created by, 50; premenopause and, 4, 12, 166; progesterone to balance, 67–68; symptoms and conditions, 48, 51–52, 67–68, 94, 202, 277–78; xenohormones and, 97

Estrogen therapy: natural, 39–40, 59, 373–74; prescribed for premenopause, 11; progesterone for women using unopposed, 371; progesterone with, 59; side effects, 5; synthetic (Premarin), 39, 59, 87, 108, 110

Estrone, 27, 49, 250, 257

European mistletoe, 45

Evening primrose oil, 153, 154, 187, 334

Exercise, 337–53; aerobic, 12–13, 342–43; benefits, 340–42; fatigue from, 9, 168, 200; heavy, and anovulation, 54; movement, 353; poses for relaxation, 352; stretching, 349–52; target heart rate, 345; walking, 344–45; weight–lifting (strength training), 12, 347–49

Eyes, dry, 51, 52, 79

Fat, body: estrogen effects, 67, 84, 95; positive aspects, 201, 285; progesterone effects, 67

Fat, dietary. *See* Essential fatty acids (EFAs); Diet and nutrition

Fatigue, 3, 4, 9, 19, 270; adrenals, tired, 163–72; estrogen

dominance and, 48, 51, 55; PMS and, 144; progestin and, 78; thyroid and, 207; xenohormones and, 97

Feet, cold, 4, 51, 52, 207, 270

Fibrocystic breasts. *See* Breasts

Fibroid tumors, 3, 4, 105–8; case history, 106–8; estrogen dominance and, 51, 110; healing recommendations, 112; hysterectomy for, 19; progesterone cream to treat, 62, 108, 111, 185, 368; surgical removal, 19, 110–11; what to avoid, 112

Flax seed oil, 154

Fluoride, 35

Folic acid, 12, 62, 223, 326–27

Follicle stimulating hormone (FSH), 12, 136–37, 192

Formby, B., 247

Gallbladder disease, 51, 56, 110, 222

Glutamine, 321

Glutathione, 223

Grant, Ellen, 156, 189, 215, 219–23, 332

Hair: coarse, 207; facial, growth of, 24; graying, 9; lip growth, 135; loss, 51, 135, 210–11; loss to arms, 85

Hands, cold, 4, 51, 53, 207, 271

Hargrove, Joel T., 147

Headaches (and migraine headaches), 194–95; alcohol and, 9; birth control pills and, 221; estrogen dominance and, 51, 56,

Headaches (*cont.*)
125, 194; healing, 195; HRT
and, 11; PMS and, 144–45;
premenopausal, 4, 10–12;
progesterone cream to treat, 62,
194, 195, 370; warding off
migraine, 194; xenohormones
and, 53

Heart health: aspirin, drawbacks,
153; attacks, progestin and,
80–81; birth control pills and,
221; estrogen and, 67–68; HRT
and, 109; magnesium and, 50;
progesterone effects, 67

Herbs, 40; adrenal-supporting, 171;
cramping formula, 115;
endometriosis, 215; for estrogen
deficiency, 59; liver-supporting
and detoxifying formula, 112,
143, 161, 181; irregular or
absent menses, 187–88; ovary-
healing, 143; PMS formula, 161;
spotting or early menses,
187–88; uterus healing formula,
112; women's formula, 181

Herman-Giddens, M. E., 95

HMOs (health maintenance
organization), 5

Hormone replacement therapy
(HRT): first attempts and uterine
cancer, 109; libido, loss of, and,
12; lupus and, 198; PMS and,
146; post-hysterectomy, 14–16,
55–56; for premenopause, 11;
progesterone supplementation,
369; unopposed estrogen,
banning, 257, 259

Hormones: across your life span, 9;
aging and, 29, 178–79; balance,

factors in, 25–29, 175; emotions,
effect on, 29; level testing,
357–60; as messengers, 30–37;
pathways, 28; synthetic, 24

Hot flashes, 17, 30, 58, 59, 63

Hrushesky, William, 183, 235

Hypoglycemia, 51

Hysterectomy, 5; birth control pills
and, 223; cervical dysplasia and,
11–12, 179; economics of, 110;
estrogen dominance and, 55–56;
fibroids and, 107–8; heavy
bleeding and, 115–16; ovarian
cysts and, 14–15; progesterone
supplementation for women with
ovaries but without a uterus,
371; unopposed estrogen and,
108–10

Immune function, 222

Infertility, 4, 188–94; adrenal
insufficiency, 165; birth control
pills and, 223; case history,
19–21; causes, 188–89;
epidemic, 55; estrogen
dominance and, 51, 55, 192;
healing, 193–94; hormone
imbalance and, 29; opportunity
for conception, 141; ovulation,
restoring, 142–43; progesterone
cream to treat, 62, 191, 192–93;
Vitex for, 193. 194; what to
avoid, 194; xenohormones and,
97

Inoh, A., 244–46

Insulin: hormone balance and, 28;
resistance, 32, 135

Iron: health risks, 35;
supplementing, 115, 334

Jacobson, J. L., 95
Jeffries, William McK., 381
Journal, daily, 12, 46–47, 127, 159, 271–72

Klausner, Richard D., 253

Leaky gut, 321
Leis, H. P., 244
Licorice, 45
Lifestyle changes, 17, 58, 128, 176–77. *See also* Premenopause Balance Program
Liver: acetaminophen and, 223; cancer, 222; estrogen dominance and, 58; hormone balance and, 28; pesticides and, 223
Lupron, 107, 147, 148
Lupus erythematosis, 98, 198
Luteinizing hormone (LH), 29; failure, 98; low levels, women affected by, 29; xenohormones and, 94, 133

Magnesium: deficiency, 50, 52, 156, 166, 194, 223; hormone balance and, 28; supplement, 187, 194, 332
Manganese, 223, 332–33
Marker, Russell E., 40
Medications: anti-inflammatory drugs (NSAIDs), 105; hormone balance and, 28; personality altering, 5
Menopause: case history, early menopause, 281–83; causes, 133–34; emotional and spiritual power, 10; fall of estrogen levels, 66; fall of progesterone levels, 66; positive aspects, 6–8
Menstruation: amenorrhea (lack of), 75–78, 271; anovulation and, 53, 134, 146, 167, 190, 366; bleeding between periods, 4, 5, 14; cramps and pain (dysmenorrhea), 24, 104, 144; cramps, mid-cycle, 14; days of, 65; early onset, 51; flooding, clotting, cramping, 113–15; healing for flooding, clotting cramping, 115; healing for irregular bleeding, 187–88; heavy bleeding, 4, 9, 19, 185–88; irregular, 3, 52, 55, 62, 168, 182–85, 270; light bleeding, 4, 9; NSAIDs and, 186; overexposure to estrogen and, 114; progesterone cream for, 186; sacredness, 158; what to avoid, 187–88
Mental acuity: estrogen and, 29; foggy thinking, 4, 201; memory loss, 4, 52, 63, 64, 165, 207; progesterone cream and, 62
Metabolism, sluggish, 52, 168
Miscarriage, 4, 190
Mitochondria, 208–9
Miyagawa, K., 80
Mohr, P. E., 237
Mood: fluctuating, 9, 52, 156; irritable, 3, 4, 24, 52, 201; PMS and, 144–45; progesterone cream to treat, 62; progestin and, 78. *See also* Depression
Muscles: pain, 79, 156–57; strain, 9; wasting, 165
Myss, Caroline, 177

Nausea and vomiting, 156
New Our Bodies, Ourselves, The
(Boston Women's Health Book
Collective), 224–25
Nicotinamide adenine dinucleoide
(NADH), 209
Night sweats, 14, 61, 62, 64
Northrup, Christiane, 177
Nutrition. *See* Diet and nutrition

Oral contraceptives. *See* Birth
control pill
Osteoporosis, 217–18; birth control
pills and, 222–23; estrogen
dominance and, 51; HRT and,
109; progesterone to prevent, 33,
217–18; strength–training,
347–49; stress and cortisol as
causal factor, 28; xenohormones
and, 97
Our Stolen Future (Colburn), 94
Ovaries, 125–43, *131, 132*; aging
and, 133–35, 178–79; awareness
of, increasing, 140–42; cancer,
129–30, 192, 219, 262–65; case
history, ovarian cyst, 125–27;
cysts, 13–17, 51, 125–27,
136–37, 138, 183, 185, 222,
262–63; emotional impact on,
138–39; follicle, 131–32, 136;
follicle damage by
xenohormones, 94; follicle
failure, 55; healing, 142;
hormone production of, over
lifetime, 135–36, 139–40;
ovulation, 53, 133, 140–42, 366;
ovulation, restoring, 142–43;
progesterone supplementation for
women without ovaries, 370–71;

removal (oophorectomy), 15,
128–30, 222; suppressed, 16;
symptoms of functional cyst,
138; what to avoid, 143, 264
Ovulation method (of birth
control), 224

Pain: abdominal, severe, 71; joint
and muscle, 79, 155–57; pelvic,
113–15, 125, 136, 185, 263. *See
also* Menstruation, cramps
Parkinson's disease, 209
Pauling, Linus, 328
PEPI (postmenopausal
estrogen/progestin intervention),
261
Phytohormones/phytoestrogens,
40–41, 45. *See also* Diet and
nutrition, soy
PMS (premenstrual syndrome), 3,
4, 144–62; diet and, 150,
155–57; emotional side of,
157–60, 215; essential fatty acids
and, 153–55; estrogen
dominance and, 51, 52–53, 55;
healing, 161–62; progesterone
cream to treat, 62, 63, 146, 148,
149, 369–70; stress, 146,
150–52; symptoms, common,
145; what to avoid, 161–62;
xenohormones and, 97
Potassium deficiency, 166
Pregnancy, 103; failure of, 135;
progesterone effects, 67, 190;
progestin, 81; prolactin, 152;
xenohormones and, 94–95, 96
Pregnenolone, 25, 377–78
Premarin. *See* Estrogen therapy
Premenopause, 3–5; age of onset, 3,

4; age for treatment, preventative, 176–78; case history, fibroid and infertility, 19–22; case history, multiple symptoms, 173–75; case history, ovarian cysts and need for balanced life, 13–17; case history, synthetic estrogen and cervical dysplasia, 9–13; case history, weight gain, 197–98; creating a positive cycle, 8–13; estrogen dominance and, 55; hormone levels in, 30–32; symptoms, 3, 4, 9, 46–47, 53, 55, 173–76; treatment, progesterone cream, 62–65; treatment guidelines for premenopausal women who are menstruating but not ovulating, 364–67; weight gain, 199–203

Premenopause Balance Program, 13, 269–384. *See also* Balance, restoring and maintaining; Diet and nutrition; Exercise; Premenopause Supplement Program; Progesterone supplementation

Premenopause Supplement Program, 322–36; minerals, 329–30; other supplements, 334–35; vitamins, 323–30

Progesterone, 25, 66–83, *79*; anovulatory cycles and, 52–54, 104, 366; body's creation of, 26–27; bone growth and, 33; breast cancer protector, 67, 234–37, *238*, *239*, 243, 244–45, 250, 258; comparison with progestin, 38–41, 82–83; conversion of diosgenin to, *41*,

40–41; days of menstrual cycle and, *65*; deficiency and premenopause, 4, 12, 13, 20, 183; estrogen dominance and need for, 50–51; excess, 36, 74, 76; molecular structure, *79*; precursor of other hormones, 27, 64, 68, 72; pregnancy and fertility, 72; receptors, 33, 68, 69; research, John Lee's, 97; roles in body, 69–73, *69*

Progesterone supplementation, 20; benefits and conditions treated, 29, 58, 61–66, 108, 168–69, 175, 178–79, 186–87, 187–88, 191, 192–93, 199, 214, 250, 257, 262; breast tenderness with initial usage, 37; dose, finding right, 74, 146, 360–64; guidelines for cream application, 362–64; guidelines for premenopausal women who are menstruating but not ovulating, 364–67; guidelines for premenopausal women who have had a hysterectomy or ovariectomy, 370–71; guidelines for women with breast fibrocysts, 368; guidelines for women with endometriosis, 367–68; guidelines for women using estrogen supplements, 368–69; guidelines for women with menstrual migraine, 370; guidelines for women with PMS, 369–70; guidelines for women with uterine fibroids, 367–68; hormone level testing, 357–60; how to use, 354–71; oral therapy,

Progesterone supplementation (*cont.*)
76, 147, 354–57; ovulation,
restoring with, 143; PMS and,
147–48, 149; resource list,
391–96; safety, 76; source of, 38;
testimonial, 62–65; transdermal
application, 243, 258, 354–57;
wild yam scam, 42–44

Progestin, synthetic (Provera),
76–83; birth control pill, 24;
breast cancer and, 244, 250, 257;
case history, birth control
implant, 76–78; characteristics
of, 24; natural versus, 38–41,
82–83; Nortestosterone, 79;
prescribed for irregular bleeding,
184; prescribed for
premenopause, 11; problems
with, 34, 60, 78–83,108 –10;
research and, 55–60; side effects,
79

Prolactin, 151–53; prolactinemia or
prolactinoma, 98

Prostaglandins, 153–55, 300

Prostate cancer, 52, 68, 233, 262

Provera. *See* Progestin, synthetic

Puberty, precocious, 95

Quercetin, 336

Rashes, 78

Rodriquez, C., 264

Safe Uses of Cortisone (Jeffries), 381

Saliva hormone test, 30, 67, 190,
239, 358

Salt, 170, 171

Sarsaparilla, 45

Schmidt, Peter J., 147

Selenium, 333, 335

Serotonin, 223

Sex: drive (libido), loss of, 3, 9, 12,
51, 63–64, 68, 95, 128, 210,
222; progesterone cream and
restoration of libido, 64

Sheehy, Gail, 109

Silent Passage, The (Sheehy), 109

Sinus problems, 52, 222

Skin: dry, 3, 79, 207; pigmentation,
167; rosacea, rashes, dermatitis,
211; thinning or papery, 165

Sleep: deprivation, 20; insomnia,
48, 52, 55, 63; need for,
increased, 9; progesterone cream
to treat disorders, 62; restless, 9;
xenohormones and, 94–95

Smith, Margaret, 149

Stress: anovulation and, 54, 365;
chronic, and hormone balance,
28–29, 30 ,163–72, 358–60;
emotional, 54; PMS and, 145,
150–53, 162; unable to cope,
168

Sweets and sugar, 172, 188, 196,
201, 271, 294–99

Tamoxifen, 245, 250–53

Testosterone, 25, 27, 64–65, 210;
deficiency, men, 29; emotions
and, 29; high, women, 30;
supplements, 381–84

Thyroid dysfunction, 203–8;
adrenals and, 169, 171; cancer,
211; case history, 203–5; cold as
symptom, 271, 278; estrogen
dominance and, 51, 67, 206;
hormone balance and, 28;
irregular periods and, 183; PMS

and, 152; progesterone effects, 67–68, 206; symptoms, 205, 206–7; treatment, 208

Urinary tract problems, 58, 59, 222
Uterus, 103–4; cancer, 51, 52, 98, 105, 109, 251–52, 253, 259–61; case history, 105–9; enlargement and fibroids, 105–8; healing recommendations, 112; keeping, 103–16; what to avoid, 112

Vaginal: dryness, 9, 58, 59, 210; mucus, 141–42
Vanadyl sulfate, 333
Vision. loss of near, 9
Vitamins: A, 11, 325; B complex, 50, 223, 325–27; B$_6$, 28, 62, 156, 187, 215, 223, 326; B$_{12}$, 12, 215, 326; C, 287, 301, 328, 335; D, 328; E, 180, 301, 329, 335; -mineral supplement, 161, 171, 180, 329–34
Vitex (chaste tree), 45, 143, 184, 193

Water retention: cortisol and, 37, 167; estrogen dominance and, 48, 52, 56, 67, 95, 125, 202; PMS and, 144–45, 148–49; progesterone effects, 67; progestin and, 79; unopposed estrogen (HRT) and, 110, 128; xenohormones and, 98
Weight: breast cancer risk and, 139; excess in stomach and hips, 19, 51, 84, 95; gain, 3, 4, 9, 11, 30, 79, 110, 140, 144, 149, 151,

165, 186–87, 199–203, 207, 286; loss, after seventy, 140; protruding belly, 135
Wild yam (diosgenin), 39, 42–44
Wiley, T. S., 247
Wolk, Alicja, 301
Women: balanced lives, 13–17, 269–83; disconnected from cycles and rhythms of body, 4; responsibility for life, 18–22; self-care and need for selfishness, 4, 18–22, 127, 159, 178, 253–54, 273–78; strategies for staying more centered, 275–77
What Your Doctor May Not Tell You about Menopause (Lee), 22, 42, 63, 192, 205, 218, 227

Xenohormones, 46, 53–56, 84–100; animals affected by, 92, 93, 98, 189–90; case history, pesticides, 84–85; comparison of, with estradiol, 91; DES, 93, 189; effects on body, 90, 97, 250; health problems in women, 98–99, 190; infertility and, 133, 190; menstrual problems and, 113–16; progesterone cream for, 176; solvents, 86–89; sources, 86–87, 303–5; techniques for decreasing exposure, 98–100

Yeast infections (candidiasis), 196–98, 319–21

Zava, David, 33, 37, 44, 66, 76, 135, 178–79, 235, 307
Zinc: deficiency, 50, 52, 67, 154, 156, 214–17; progesterone effects, 66; supplement, 334

About the Authors

❖

John R. Lee, M.D. (1929–2003), is internationally acknowledged as a pioneer and expert in the study and use of the hormone progesterone, and on the subject of hormone replacement therapy for women. He used transdermal progesterone extensively in his clinical practice for nearly a decade, doing research that showed that it can reverse osteoporosis. Dr. Lee had a distinguished medical career, including graduating from Harvard and the University of Minnesota Medical School. He retired from a 30-year family practice in Northern California and began writing and traveling around the world speaking to doctors, scientists, and laypeople about progesterone. Dr. Lee taught a very popular course on Optimal Health at the College of Marin for 15 years. He is the author of *Optimal Health Guidelines*, *Natural Progesterone: The Multiple Roles of a Remarkable Hormone* (written for doctors) and the best-sellers *What Your Doctor May Not Tell You About Menopause*, *What Your Doctor May Not Tell You About Premenopause*, and *What*

Your Doctor May Not *Tell You About Breast Cancer* and was editor-in-chief of the *John R. Lee, M.D., Medical Letter.*

Jesse Lynn Hanley, M.D., entered medical school at the University of Illinois, Chicago, at the age of twenty-nine, inspired by her own recovery from chronic illness with natural methods. Having been a masseuse, yogi, vegetarian, and student of nutrition and psychotherapy prior to entering medical school, her perspective was naturally more encompassing than most. During medical school she simultaneously began her study of oriental medicine and acupuncture at UCLA Medical School, integrating both models along the way with her in-depth nutrition knowledge. Of the past fourteen years of private practice, her last seven have been as medical director of Malibu Health Center and now Malibu Health and Rehabilitation. She has been recognized on several occasions for her outstanding contributions to the holistic medical community and was the health expert on *Wake Up America* for KFOX radio. Dr. Hanley was the associate editor of *Malibu Health Styles Newsletter*, writing a monthly column. She lectures to other physicians and the public on numerous health topics and is currently the president of the Malibu Medical Society. Dr. Hanley's philosophy as medical director of a multidisciplinary wellness center in Malibu, California, is to accentuate the person's/patient's empowerment with education and support systems, and to develop personalized health care programs.

Virginia Hopkins, M.A., has been a writer and editor since she graduated from Yale University in 1976. She has a master's degree in applied psychology from the University of Santa Monica. She is the coauthor, with John R. Lee, M.D., of *What Your Doctor May* Not *Tell You About Menopause: The Breakthrough Book on Natural Progesterone* (Warner Books, 1996), *What Your Doctor May* Not *Tell You About Premenopause* (Warner Books, 1999), *What Your Doctor May* Not *Tell You About Breast Cancer* (Warner Books, 2003), and *Prescription Alternatives* (Keats Publishing, 1998), which she coauthored with Earl Mindell, R.Ph., Ph.D. She was the executive editor of the *John R. Lee, M.D., Medical Letter,* and has written or coauthored more than 30 books on alternative health and nutrition.

FIBROMYALGIA
The Revolutionary Treatment That Can
Reverse the Disease

FIBROMYALGIA FATIGUE
The Powerful Program That Helps You Boost
Your Energy and Reclaim Your Life

GLAUCOMA
The Essential Treatments and Advances That
Could Save Your Sight

HIP AND KNEE REPLACEMENT SURGERY
Everything You Need to Know to
Make the Right Decisions

HPV AND ABNORMAL PAP SMEARS
Get the Facts on This Dangerous Virus—
Protect Your Health and Your Life!

HYPERTENSION
The Revolutionary Nutrition and Lifestyle
Program toHelp Fight High Blood Pressure

HYPOTHYROIDISM
A Simple Plan for Extraordinary Results

IBS
Eliminate Your Symptoms and Live a
Pain-free, Drug-free Life

more...

KNEE PAIN AND SURGERY
Learn the Truth About MRIs and Common
Misdiagnoses—and Avoid Unnecessary Surgery

MENOPAUSE
The Breakthrough Book on *Natural* Hormone Balance

MIGRAINES
The Breakthrough Program That Can
Help End Your Pain

OSTEOPOROSIS
Help Prevent—and Even Reverse—the Disease
That Burdens Millions of Women

PARKINSON'S DISEASE
A Holistic Program for Optimal Wellness

PEDIATRIC FIBROMYALGIA
A Safe, New Treatment Plan for Children

PREMENOPAUSE
Balance Your Hormones and Your Life
from Thirty to Fifty

PROSTATE CANCER
The Breakthrough Information and TreatmentsThat
Can Help Save Your Life

SINUSITUS
Relieve Your Symptoms and Identify the
Real Source of Your Pain